PROSTATE CANCER
QUESTIONS AND ANSWERS

A. COLIN BUCK

Dedicated to Geoffrey Chisholm, friend and mentor

PUBLISHING INTERNATIONAL

© 1995 All rights reserved. No part of this publication may be reproduced, stored in a retrieval system or transmitted in any form or by any means, electronic, mechanical, photocopying, recording or otherwise, without the prior permission of the copyright owner.

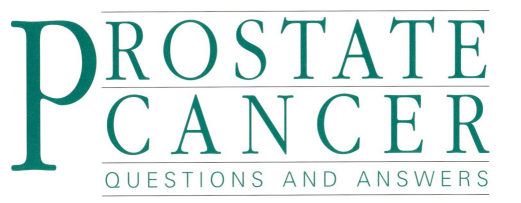

PROSTATE CANCER
QUESTIONS AND ANSWERS

Published by:

MERIT PUBLISHING INTERNATIONAL

European address:
35 Winchester Street
Basingstoke
Hampshire RG21 1EE
England

North American address:
8260 NW 49th Manor
Pine Grove
Coral Springs, Florida,
33067 U.S.A.

ISBN 1 873413 85 8

A. COLIN BUCK

Consultant Urologist, Glasgow Royal Infirmary

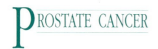

CONTENTS

Foreword   5
by William R. Fair

Chapter 1   9
Epidemiology of prostate cancer

Chapter 2   21
Clinical presentation, investigation and diagnosis

Chapter 3   47
Pathology of prostate cancer

Chapter 4   55
Clinical management of prostate cancer

Chapter 5   87
The treatment of hormone-escaped disease
by Colin Buck and Dermott Lanigan

Chapter 6   93
Screening for prostate cancer

Chapter 7   99
Questions commonly asked by patients
by Dermott Lanigan

References   105

Acknowledgements   109

FOREWORD

This book by Colin Buck provides a practical, up-to-date guide on prostate cancer which addresses the concerns most frequently expressed by patients and referring physicians. Along with a review of the natural history, epidemiology and pathology of the disease, it includes a comprehensive discussion of clinical issues concerning diagnosis and therapy.

The author considers the treatment of both localized and metastatic disease in a format that will provide the practitioner with authoritative answers to questions commonly posed by patients with prostatic cancer and their families. The section on controversies in the management of prostatic cancer is particularly informative and should be helpful to all those dealing with this often confusing and controversial disease.

Mr. Buck brings a wealth of clinical experience to this task, and has produced a volume that I predict will be widely utilized by urologists, medical oncologists, radiation oncologists, general practitioners, and patients faced with the sometimes overwhelming task of finding the right path in the management of prostatic cancer.

WILLIAM R. FAIR
Chief, Urologic Surgery
Florence and Theodore Baumritter/Enid Ancell Chair of Urologic Oncology
Memorial Sloane-Kettering Cancer Center
New York City, N.Y.

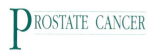

PROSTATE CANCER
QUESTIONS AND ANSWERS

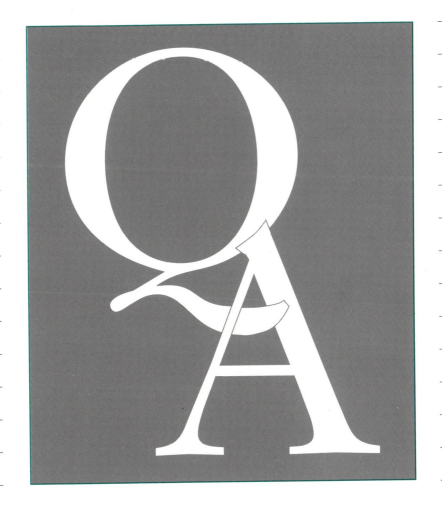

A. COLIN BUCK

merit
PUBLISHING
INTERNATIONAL

CHAPTER ONE

EPIDEMIOLOGY

How common is prostate cancer?

Introduction
Cancer of the prostate is the second or third most common malignancy in western industrialized countries and the fifth most commonly diagnosed cancer in the world. In the United States, prostatic cancer is now the most commonly diagnosed cancer and the second most common cause of death from malignant disease in men, after cancer of the lung (Figure 1).

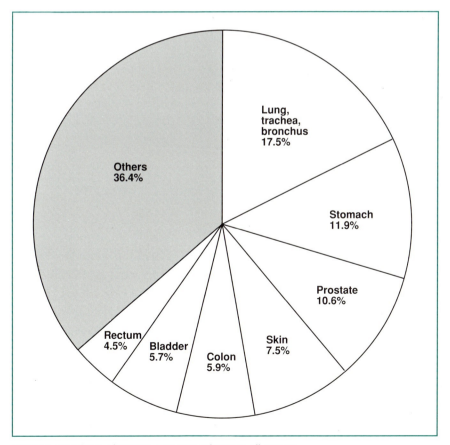

Figure 1. *Incidence of prostate cancer in relation to all cancers.*

PROSTATE CANCER

It is estimated that in 1994 approximately 165,000 new cases of prostatic cancer will be diagnosed in the United States and nearly 35,000 men will die from it.

In 1992, the disease claimed 9,629 lives in the United Kingdom, more than four times as many as cervical cancer. Based on the UN population projections, Peter Boyle, director of the Division of Epidemiology and Biostatistics at the European Institute of Oncology in Milan, predicts that the number of prostate cancer cases will double in Europe over the next 20–30 years, continuing the upward trend of recent decades.

Furthermore, autopsy studies have shown that 30% of men over 50 years of age have histologic evidence of so-called latent prostatic cancer, disease that remains undetected during the patient's lifetime (Franks, 1973). The incidence steadily increases with age, ranging from 10% in men in their 50s to 80% in men in their 80s; thus, every decade of ageing nearly doubles the incidence. It is clear, therefore, that the prevalence of prostate cancer seen on autopsy examination far outstrips the prevalence of clinical cancer. Curiously, and unique to the prostate, only about a tenth of these latent cancers will become clinically manifest during the patient's lifetime; thus, nine of ten such cancers do not seem to matter.

Although clinical prostate cancer can and does occur in men in their 40s, approximately 85% of prostate cancer patients are over 65 years of age (Figure 2).

Has there been a genuine increase in the incidence of prostate cancer?

Over the past 15 to 20 years there has been a steady increase in the reported incidence of prostate cancer in most parts of the world for which statistics are available. For example, in the USA the age-adjusted incidence of prostate cancer in 1973 was 105.1 for blacks and 62.4 for whites. In 1987, the incidence figures were 136.1 and 99.2 respectively (Table 1). Even within one country, (the USA) the incidence rates vary considerably. Recent data (1988) show that the age-adjusted incidence in Minnesota men was 114.7 per 100,000 while among men in Seattle it was 158.6 per 100,000.

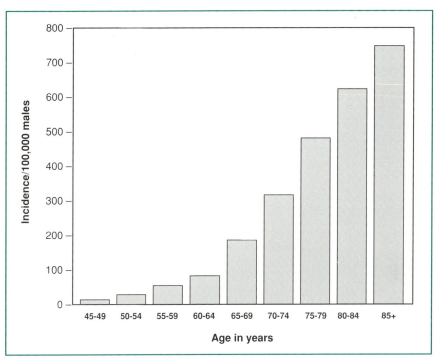

Figure 2. *Prostate cancer is virtually unknown in men aged below 45 years, but the incidence increases with age. 85% of prostate cancer patients are over 65 years. Although the peak age for new diagnoses is about 70 years, the age incidence continues to rise. This is because there are fewer men, at risk, due to death from other causes. Also the proportion of elderly men in the population is increasing.*

Three important factors underlie the apparently increasing rates of prostatic cancer:

Population changes
Between 1970 and 1987 there was a 68% increase in the male population aged 75–84 years and a 100% increase in the number of men over the age of 85 (Figure 3). Clearly, the population of men at risk from prostatic cancer has increased.

Screening
The trend towards screening 'at-risk' populations, particularly in the USA, will undoubtedly uncover the very large pool of latent cancers and substantially change the apparent incidence of the disease.

Prostate Cancer

Table 1. *Age-adjusted incidence of prostatic cancer, according to the year of diagnosis.*

RACE	INCIDENCE OF PROSTATIC CANCER ‡						
	1973	1974	1975	1976	1977	1978	1979	1980
	Number of cases per 100,000 population						
BLACK	105.1	99.2	110.7	109.3	121.3	115.9	122.7	125.5
WHITE	62.4	64.5	68.5	72.2	73.9	72.8	76.3	78.0
	1981	1982	1983	1984	1985	1986	1987
	Number of cases per 100,000 population						
BLACK	125.7	129.1	131.0	136.4	130.2	126.8	136.1
WHITE	80.1	80.3	83.3	82.0	85.7	89.1	99.2

‡Age adjusted to the 1970 U.S. standard population

Data obtained from the National Cancer Institute Surveillance Epidemiology and End-Results Program

Incidental diagnosis

With a larger and healthier elderly male population and improved surgical techniques there has been a substantial increase in surgery for benign prostate disease with a concomitant increase in the diagnosis of incidental carcinomas.

The fact that prostate cancer mortalities have not changed in parallel with the increased incidence suggests that no genuine change has taken place in the disease or its risk factors and that variations in the detection of prostate cancer, rather than its occurrence, are responsible for the apparent increase in incidence (Figure 4).

Are there any causative or predisposing risk factors for prostate cancer?

Epidemiologic studies suggest a correlation between prostate cancer and certain risk factors:

Genetic factors

The unique predilection of prostate cancer for the human species, the differing incidence and mortalities around the world, its changing rate as

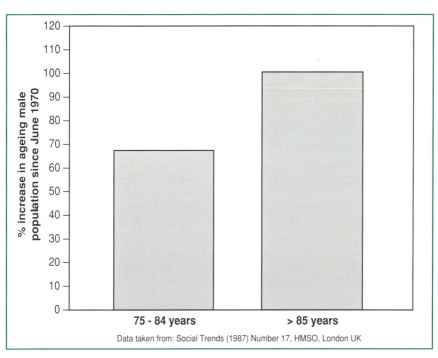

Figure 3. *Increase in ageing male population from 1970 – 1987.*

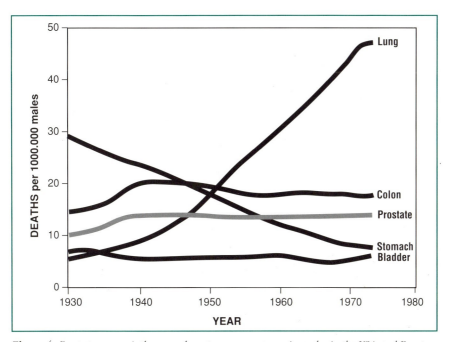

Figure 4. *Prostate cancer is the second most common cancer in males in the USA and Europe. It accounts for approximately 10% of all cancer deaths in males and this death rate has remained almost steady over the past 40 years (unlike that for lung cancer, which has increased and for stomach and colorectal cancer, which have decreased).*

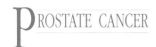

man moves from a low-risk area to a high-risk area and its variable pattern within a population, appear not to support an etiologic role for genetic factors. Nevertheless, there is a higher incidence of cancer among relatives of patients with prostatic cancer. More significantly, when cancer occurs in a patient with an affected first-degree relative (father or brother) and/or a second-degree relative (uncle or grandfather) there is an eight-fold increase in risk. In these family clusters the disease develops at an earlier age and appears to run a more aggressive course, suggesting that genetic factors influence the biological behavior of the tumor.

Interestingly, a recent study from Iceland has shown that the risk of prostate cancer was significantly raised for all first degree (1.4) and second degree (1.3) relatives of women with breast cancer and that the risk of prostate cancer was further raised if the proband with breast cancer had a first degree relative with prostate cancer (Tulinius et al., 1992).

Although these features argue for a genetic inheritance of susceptibility any such phenomenon are actually determined by genetic and environmental factors at the same time. A proper definition of genetic determination, therefore, should not refer to features of individual organisms, but rather to differences in features between organisms. Such differences may be genetic in the sense that they are due only to a genetic difference, not an environmental one. Therefore, a feature can be genetic under one comparison and environmental (or more correctly genetic and environmental) under a different comparison.

There is much variation in populations. Part of it can be attributed to genetic causes, another part to environmental causes. Statements concerning a particular population (i.e. Iceland) need not permit generalizations. The contribution of genetic factors to the variation in some features may be very different in different populations. Iceland has one of the most genetically homogenous populations in the world, thus aetiologies concerning genetics may be context dependent.

Context dependence is an important pitfall in the search for genetic causes of a disease, but it is not the only one. Suppose we know that all patients suffering from a particular disorder have one allele of some gene, whereas all healthy persons have a different allele. Suppose further that there are no other systemic genetic differences between the two groups. Would this justify the conclusion that the presence of clinical characteristics of the disease and an absence of these features is due to a difference in the gene? At first sight, yes. But there is no warrant for it. The reason is that there may be systematic environmental differences as well. In the Icelandic population the assumption that the disease is genetically determined is actually weakened - environmental factors seem to be, at least, aggravating to a far greater degree.

So far no specific chromosomal markers or deletions have been identified in prostate cancer. This is an area of research that is generating considerable interest.

Geographic and racial factors
There are well recognized geographic and racial differences in the incidence of, and mortality from, prostatic cancer. The incidence is highest in the Afro-American population, with 136.1 cases per 100,000 in Almeida County blacks. This is significantly higher than whites in America who have an incidence of 99.2 per 100,000 (1987). Ross et al. (1986) have shown that young adult black men have circulating testosterone concentrations 10–15% higher than in young adult white men, which may relate to the underlying differences in subsequent prostate cancer incidence between the two populations.

The lowest incidence of prostatic cancer is seen in the Far East. Among the Japanese, the incidence is 3.4 per 100,000 of the population, and in China it is only 0.8 per 100,000 of the population. There are no significant differences between the serum testosterone concentrations of young adult Japanese men and of young adult white or black men (Japanese values are intermediate between the whites and the blacks) (Figure 5).

However, Japanese men were found to have significantly reduced sex hormone binding globulin (SHBG) levels and reduced 5 α reductase activity compared with the other two groups. (Ross et al., 1992). Schroder compared plasma testosterone levels in 368 Dutch men and 258 Japanese and found a significantly lower plasma testosterone level in the Japanese.

It is important in this context to take into account that five cases of prostate cancer occurring at an unusually early age have been recorded in body-builders using anabolic steroids. The diagnosis was made in the youngest of these at only 40 years of age (Roberts and Essenhigh, 1986).

PROSTATE CANCER

The use and abuse of anabolic steroids is becoming increasingly commonplace and their use among weight-lifters and body-builders is estimated to be as high as 80%. These drugs will enjoy continued popularity among athletes until their long-term and life-threatening effects are better publicized.

Prostate cancer is more prevalent in Northern Europe and North America than in Latin America and Southern Europe. However, most autopsy studies suggest that the prevalence of latent cancer is the same for all races in almost all countries.

When people migrate from an area of low incidence of prostate cancer to one of high incidence, for example when Japanese and European men emigrate to the United States, protection seems to last for one generation before the incidence begins to rise.

Environmental factors

Mortality from prostate cancer appears to be increased among men living

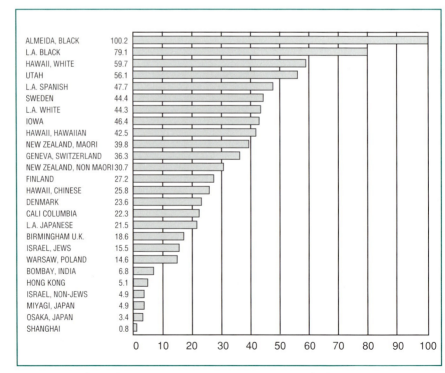

Figure 5. *Incidence of prostate cancer among various regions and ethnic groups.*

in urban areas where exposure to environmental pollution with automobile exhaust fumes, cadmium, chemical fertilizers and other industrial chemical carcinogens is higher.

Cadmium. Two small cohort studies, one of smelter workers exposed to cadmium and the other of workers exposed to cadmium oxide in various occupations, have suggested that workers exposed to cadmium may have an increased risk of prostate cancer. In the former study, by Leman et al. (1976), four deaths from prostate cancer occurred among 92 decedents versus an expected number of 1.2.

A study by Kipling and Waterhouse (1967) reported that four prostate cancers developed among 248 workers exposed to cadmium oxide for a minimum of one year, compared with only 0.6 expected. Furthermore, when Winkelstein and Kantor (1969) reported a positive correlation between prostate cancer mortality and particulate air pollution levels in Buffalo, New York, they speculated that it could be a reflection of cadmium levels in urban air.

Cigarette smoke, certain dietary items such as oysters and soft drinking water are other potential sources of cadmium (Schroeder et al., 1967). However there is little epidemiological evidence that any of these factors substantially influence prostate cancer risk.

Overall, the totality of epidemiologic evidence suggests that if cadmium is an etiologic agent for prostate cancer, only a small proportion of cases can be attributed to such exposure.

Radioactivity. The most disturbing data concerning a specific hazard for prostate cancer emerged from a study reported in 1988 by Dr Valerie Berral and her colleagues. The investigation concerned workers in the nuclear weapons and nuclear fuels' industry employed at the Sellafield plant of British Nuclear Fuels and the UK Atomic Energy Authority and the Atomic Weapons Establishment. Those employees with a documented radiation record had a rate-ratio for prostatic carcinoma of 1.9 compared with other employees and the ratio rose to 2.23 ($p<0.05$) when a 10 year time lag was added to the analysis.

Prostate Cancer

The same group has also recently reported that the risk of prostatic cancer was significantly increased in men employed by the United Kingdom Atomic Energy Authority who were occupationally exposed to (and found to be internally contaminated with) tritium, Cr51, Fe59, Co60 or Zn65 from 1946 to 1986 (Rooney et al., 1993). The relative risks increased with increasing level and duration of potential exposure to each of the radionuclides. The relative risk tended to be higher in younger men and in men whose deaths were directly attributed to prostatic cancer, suggesting that the malignancies associated with radionuclide exposure were not the relatively benign tumors sometimes diagnosed co-incidentally in old men.

Diet. There is no convincing evidence to relate prostate cancer to patterns of sexual behavior, venereal infection, any particular lifestyle, or smoking, and no etiological viral agent has yet been discovered. However, there seems to be a link with dietary animal fat.

TABLE 2. *Evidence supporting a dietary hypothesis for the cause of prostatic cancer.*

♦ A strong positive correlation between dietary fat consumption and prostate cancer incidence.

♦ Breast and prostate cancer rates are closely correlated in most countries: both are most common in the United States and in Western/Northern Europe, where fat consumption is high.

♦ Prostate cancer rates are highest in US states that have a high fat consumption.

♦ Time trends within Japan: fat intake and prostate cancer have increased steadily with time since 1950.

(Wynder et al., 1984)

Armstrong and Doll (1975), found a strong correlation between per capita consumption of dietary fat and prostate cancer mortality. It has been postulated that dietary fat affects cancer occurrence via alterations in the hormone environment (Berg, 1975).

In a case control study of 110 cases of prostate cancer, Ross et al., (1983) noted that cases consumed fewer carrots than age-matched controls. Carrot consumption is a good index of dietary vitamin A, which protects against the development of epithelial cancers, including prostate cancer (Peto et al., 1981). A western diet, high in animal fat, low in fiber, and lacking in betacarotene, is thought to be a risk factor for prostate cancer (Table 2).

Prostate Cancer

CHAPTER 2

CLINICAL PRESENTATION, INVESTIGATION AND DIAGNOSIS

How does cancer of the prostate present?

Most patients with prostate cancer present with the signs and symptoms of outflow obstruction. The urinary symptoms closely resemble those usually associated with benign prostatic hypertrophy (BPH) and indeed show few practical points of distinction. It is said that there is often a relatively shorter history (months rather than years) of urinary symptoms, but this is questionable. However, nocturnal incontinence associated with residual urine seems to be relatively more common in prostate cancer (Fergusson, 1963).

Approximately 10–15% of patients present with symptoms that relate only to their metastases, mostly pain referable to their bony deposits. Occasionally, patients themselves detect the presence of an abdominal mass or enlarged superficial inguinal glands due to lymphatic involvement, while others note edema of the lower extremeties from the same cause.

Sometimes, patients present in renal failure due to extensive local disease obstructing the ureters. More rarely, they present with spinal cord compression, anemia or cachexia. Very occasionally, advanced disease may be an incidental finding in the course of a routine examination (an appropriate term for these cases would be occult cancer).

At the time of initial presentation, about 70–80% of prostate cancer patients are found to have either locally advanced disease or distant metastases. For them, treatment can only be palliative, supportive and symptomatic. In approximately 20% of patients, the disease is localized and confined to the prostate: 10–15% of such cases are detected by histologic examination of resected prostate tissue or adenoma enucleated for BPH (incidental carcinoma of the prostate); in the remaining 5-10%, a hard nodule or suspicious induration and/or palpable distortion of the prostate contour on rectal examination leads to a biopsy-proven diagnosis.

PROSTATE CANCER

In summary, the clinical manifestations of carcinoma of the prostate are variable and unpredictable. At one end of the spectrum is a highly aggressive and malignant disease that disseminates widely and rapidly. At the other end is an indolent and slow-growing cancer that remains localized for a long period of time, producing very little in the way of signs and symptoms.

The natural histories of these tumors are very different, raising difficult questions concerning their management. Clearly, the aggressive, disseminated tumor may only be influenced by hormonal manipulation but cannot be cured, but does the low biologic potential of the others make any attempt at curative therapy meddlesome and superfluous?

How should a patient presenting with cancer of the prostate be treated?

There are two aspects to the treatment of prostatic cancer: first, relief of symptoms and, secondly, management of the cancer which, of course, depends on the stage or the extent of the disease.

In patients presenting with outflow tract obstruction, the first priority must be the relief of obstruction. Trans-urethral resection (TUR) of the prostate is still the most frequently performed operation for obstruction due to carcinoma. However, although there is no clear evidence that this operation contributes to the spread of the disease, the possibility cannot be excluded. Patients presenting with acute or chronic retention of urine will require catheterization.

Some patients with a hard, craggy gland on rectal examination, supported by a proven diagnosis on needle biopsy or aspiration cytology, will benefit from the initiation of hormonal treatment to shrink the prostate and relieve obstruction, thus obviating the need for a TUR. Endocrine therapy, whether with orchidectomy, estrogens, anti-androgens or luteinizing hormone-releasing hormone (LH-RH) analogs, leads to a volume reduction of the primary tumor by more than 50% (Figure 6).

In patients who presents with renal failure due to bilateral ureteric obstruction and hydronephrosis, there is every justification for the insertion of either unilateral or bilateral nephrostomy tubes or stents, as any subsequent hormonal treatment will shrink the primary lesion and provide worthwhile palliation for metastatic disease.

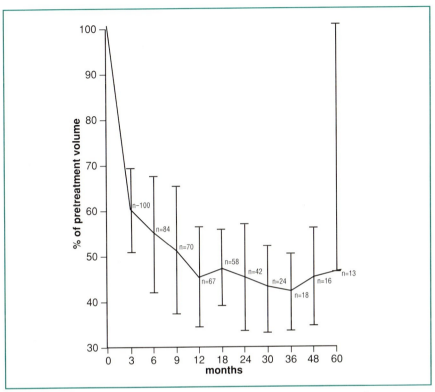

Figure 6. *Decrease in volume of the primary tumor under endocrine treatment (castration or LH-RH analog) measured in 100 patients over time. The diagram indicates average volume changes measured by transrectal ultrasonography and standard deviations of the mean.*

What are the criteria for the management of the patient with prostate cancer?

The management of carcinoma of the prostate depends upon three related factors:

- an accurate histologic diagnosis
- the pathologic grade of the tumor
- the clinical stage of the disease.

Histology

Histologic diagnosis is obligatory in prostate cancer and is obtained from histology of the TUR chips, a Trucut needle biopsy, or aspiration cytology. The advantages of the TUR and Trucut needle biopsy material are that the tissue provides information about cellular abnormalities and nuclear anaplasia as well as the stromal invasive/infiltrative characteristics of the tumor, whereas aspiration biopsy provides information only on cellular morphology.

Prostate Cancer

In the exceptional circumstances where there is overwhelming corroborative evidence for prostate cancer, such as very high levels of prostatic specific antigen (PSA) and prostatic acid phosphatase (PAP), osteoblastic metastases and a palpably hard gland together with a clinical response to androgen deprivation, the need for a histologic diagnosis may be overlooked.

Grading of prostatic carcinoma

Histologic grading of all tumors, including prostate cancer, is based on the degree of differentiation or anaplasia of tumor cells. Many pathologists simply grade prostate cancers as well, moderately, or poorly differentiated. However, approximately 50% of prostate cancers express more than one histologic pattern and unless this heterogeneity is taken into account, it is difficult to accurately relate the grade of a prostate cancer to its prognosis.

This problem was addressed in a grading system first proposed by Gleason and Mellinger in 1974. The Gleason System, which has now been adopted worldwide as the standard reference for the grading of prostatic cancer, considers the degree of differentiation of the tumor and the relationship of the glands to the stroma.

Five different histologic grades of tumor differentiation are recognized. The predominant grade present in the tumor, based on the area involved, is called the primary grade and the less representative grade is called the secondary grade (Figure 7–12). For each tumor, therefore, two grades are determined which, when added together, provide a Gleason histologic score ranging from 2 to 10.

The Gleason score appears to be a good predictor of prognosis. A strong correlation was observed between the histologic score and the presence of identifiable metastases, pain due to cancer, dilatation of the upper tract and abnormal elevation of the serum PAP (Gleason and Mellinger, 1974).

More recently, the Gleason score was reported to correlate positively with the PSA level. In one study, no patient with a Gleason score of 4 or less showed progression of disease, five of 47 patients (11%) with Gleason grade 5 and 6 progressed, and seven of 21 (33%) with scores of 7–9 progressed (Cantrell et al.,1981). There is good evidence that a patient with a low Gleason score (2–4) will not have pelvic lymph node metastases, will not develop progression of the tumor, and will have a normal life expectancy (1982; Kramer et al., 1980, Sagalowsky et al.,).

Staging of prostatic cancer

The staging of the disease is central to any decision regarding treatment, and to the prediction of outcome. It is based on an evaluation of the extent of the primary tumor, and the presence or absence of metastases. Biochemical tumor markers and advances in imaging techniques have improved the accuracy of staging.

Two main staging systems are presently in use. In the Whitmore-Jewett staging system, which is generally used in the United States, the primary tumor is denoted by four categories, A through D. The other method is the TNM classification proposed by the UICC (Tables 3a and 3b).

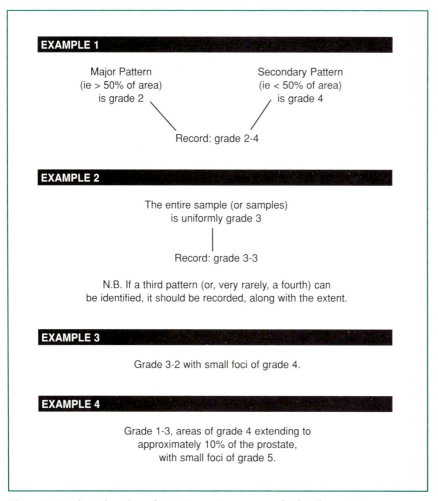

Figure 7. *Histological grading of prostatic carcinoma cancer by the Gleason System.*

PROSTATE CANCER

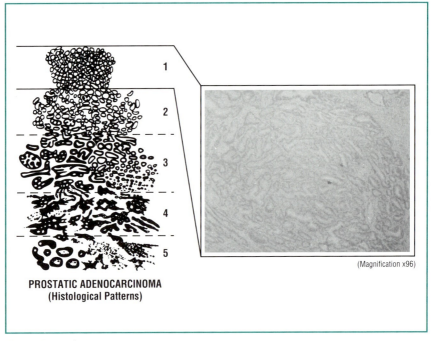

Figure 8. Grade 1.

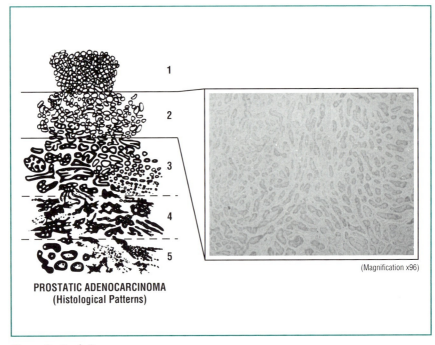

Figure 9. Grade 2.

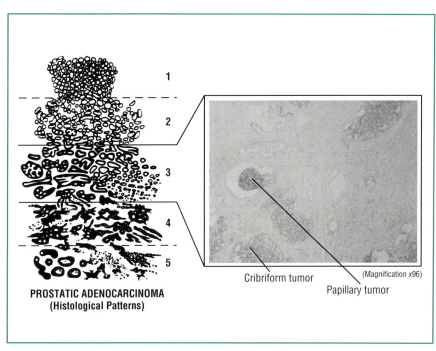

Figure 10. *Grade 3.*

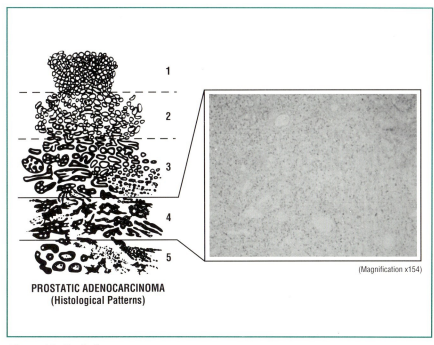

Figure 11. *Grade 4.*

PROSTATE CANCER
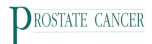

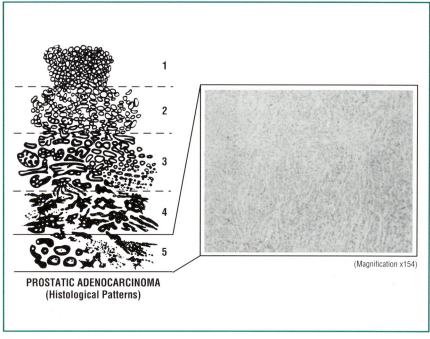

Figure 12. *Grade 5.*

Pattern	Margin of Tumor Areas	Gland Pattern	Gland Size	Gland Distribution
1	Well defined	Single, separate, round	Medium	Closely packed
2	Less defined	Single, separate, rounded, but more variable	Medium	Spaced up to one gland diameter apart, on average
3	Poorly defined	Single, separate, more irregular	Small, medium, or large	Spaced more than one gland diameter apart, rarely packed
or 3	Poorly defined	Rounded masses of cribriform or papillary epithelium	Medium or large	Rounded masses with smooth sharp edges
4	Ragged, infiltrating	Fused glandular masses or 'hypernephroid'	Small	Fused in ragged masses
5	Ragged, infiltrating	Almost absent, few tiny glands or signet ring cells	Small	Ragged anaplastic masses of epithelium
or 5	Poorly defined	Few small lumina in rounded masses of solid epithelium central necrosis?	Small	Rounded masses and cords with smooth, sharp edges

Figure 13. *Histological patterns of adenocarcinoma of the prostate.*

TABLE 3a. *Staging of prostatic cancer.*

Whitmore 1956 (with modifications) Stage		TNM 1978-82 Category		TNM 1992	
A	Not palpable on rectal exam	T0pT1-3	No tumor palpable	T0	No evidence of primary tumor
	A1 Focal cancer (< 3 chips)	T0pT1	< 3 foci	T1	Clinically inapparent tumor, not palpable and not visible by imaging
				T1a	Tumor an incidental histological finding in ≤ 5% of tissue resected
	A2 Diffuse (> 3 chips)	T0pT2 3	> 3 foci	T1b	Tumor an incidental histological finding in > 5% of tissue resected
				T1c	Tumor identified by needle biopsy (e.g. because of elevated serum PSA)
B	**B1** Unilobar, < 2 cm	T1	Tumor intracapsular; surrounded by palpable normal gland	T2	Tumor confined withing the prostate ●
				T2a	Tumor involves more than half of a lobe or less
	B2 Unilobar, > 2cm	T2	Tumor confined to gland; smooth nodule deforming contour	T2b	Tumor involves more than half a lobe but not both lobes
	B3 All other, intracapsular			T2c	Tumor involves both lobes
C	Extending through capsule	T3	Tumor extending beyond capsule with or without involvement of lateral sulci and/or seminal vesicles	T3	Tumor extends through the prostatic capsule ▲
	C1 Sulcus or sulci not free			T3a	Unilateral extracapsular extension
	C2 > Base of seminal vesicles ± sulci			T3b	Bilateral extracapsular extension
				T3c	Tumor invades seminal vesicle(s)
	C3 > Base of seminal vesicles ± other adjacent organs	T4	Tumor fixed or infiltrating neighbouring structures	T4	Tumor fixed or invades adjacent structures other than seminal vesicles
				T4a	Tumor invades bladder neck and/or external sphincter and/or rectum
				T4b	Tumor invades levator muscles and/or is fixed to pelvic wall
D	Any local extension				
	D1 Lymph node involvement				
	D2 Other metastases				

● Tumor found in one or both lobes by needle biopsy, but not palpable or visible by imaging, is classified as T1c.
▲ Invasion into the prostatic apex or into (but not beyond) the prostatic capsule is not classified as T3 but as T2.

Prostate Cancer

TABLE 3b. *Illustrated staging of prostatic cancer.*

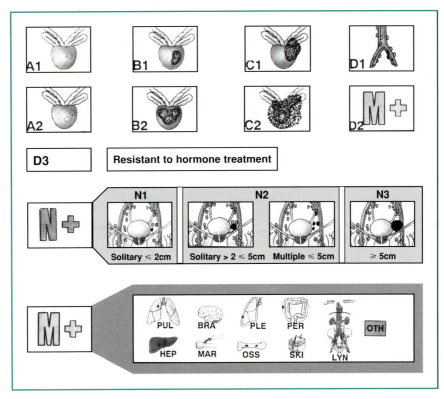

The subdivisions of the primary tumor categories in both staging systems can be confusing when trying to draw comparisons; therefore, attempts to unify the two systems have been made, leading to recent modifications of the T category.

For example, the TNM classification does not differentiate between unilobar tumors < 2 cm in diameter and larger intracapsular tumors, nor does it make any distinction between focal and multifocal disease. In the TNM classification of 1992, the T0 category now denotes 'no primary tumor' and, therefore, T1a and T1b correspond to the Jewett-Whitmore A1 and A2 categories.

How is the primary tumor assessed?

The assessment of the primary tumor is both clinical - by digital rectal examination (DRE), assisted by transrectal ultrasound (TRUS); and pathologic - by examination of the tissue obtained by TUR.

How accurate is digital rectal examination in diagnosing prostatic cancer?

It is generally agreed that DRE of the prostate is highly subjective and flawed by observer error. A gland that is extensively involved by a T3 or T4 tumor is unmistakable on rectal examination and the ability to detect these lesions doubtless increases with experience.

On the other hand, however, diagnosis by DRE is considerably more difficult when there is a subtle change in the consistency within a lobe of the gland, or when it is necessary to determine the nature of a tumor nodule distorting the contour of the prostate. Here, even the most 'educated' finger may fail, and few urologists would be entirely confident of their clinical ability. In addition, DRE cannot be used to assess the anterior and antero-lateral aspects of the prostate gland. Overall, DRE is the least accurate screening modality.

How helpful is transrectal ultrasonography in the diagnosis and assessment of the primary lesion?

Transrectal ultrasonography should be regarded as complementary to DRE. TRUS of the prostate is able to detect hypoechoic areas (which may represent a carcinoma) as small as 5 mm in diameter. It is said to detect clinically important lesions that are outside the range of the examining finger. Furthermore, it is a harmless procedure, carried out with the patient in the left lateral position with knees and hips flexed and is not painful or unpleasant when performed gently. It can be performed routinely as an office procedure by urologists or in radiology departments.

A normal prostate scan appearance is shown in Figure 14. The characteristic and most frequently observed ultrasonic appearance of prostate cancer is hypoechogenicity. In a number of studies, 65–70% of hypoechoic lesions of the prostate have proved to be malignant (Lee et al., 1986; Dahnert et al., 1986); however, some cancers may be hypoechoic (Figure 15) while others may be isoechoic (Figure 16) as was thought to be invariably the case when ultrasound imaging was first introduced.

The integrity of the capsule of the prostate can be assessed on ultrasound, and breaches and distortions of the outline indicating extracapsular extension of the carcinoma, (Figure 17) an important consideration in staging with a view to operability, can be determined.

Prostate Cancer

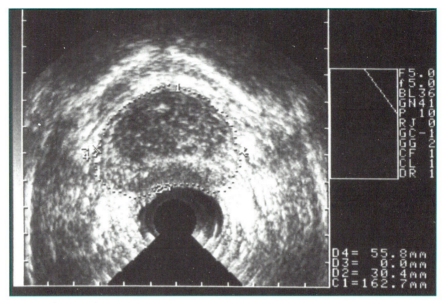

Figure 14. *Normal prostate scan.*

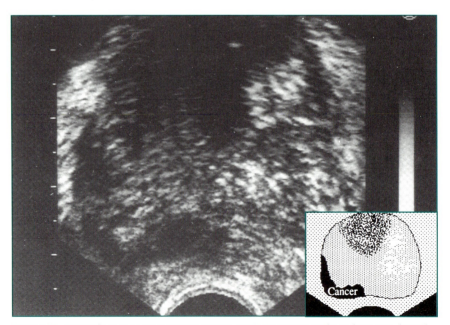

Figure 15. *Hypoechoic zone on transvers section. Prostatic cancer in the right postero-lateral region of the peripheral zone.*

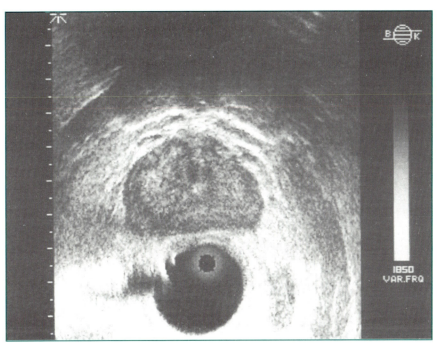

Figure 16. *Poor visualization of the craniocaudal differentitation: isoechoic type appearance. This frame shows asymmetry of the prostate gland with apparent enlargement of the right lobe. The craniocaudal differntiation is not clearly defined. The prostate gland was firm to palpation and the serum prostate specific antigen level was 47ng/ml. Multiple biopsies revealed the presence of adenocarcinoma in both lobes.*

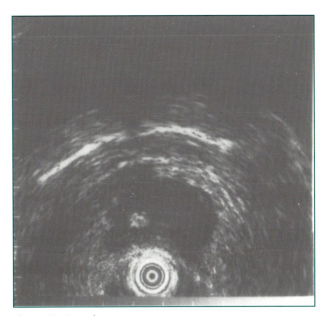

Figure 17. *Irregular prostate scan.*

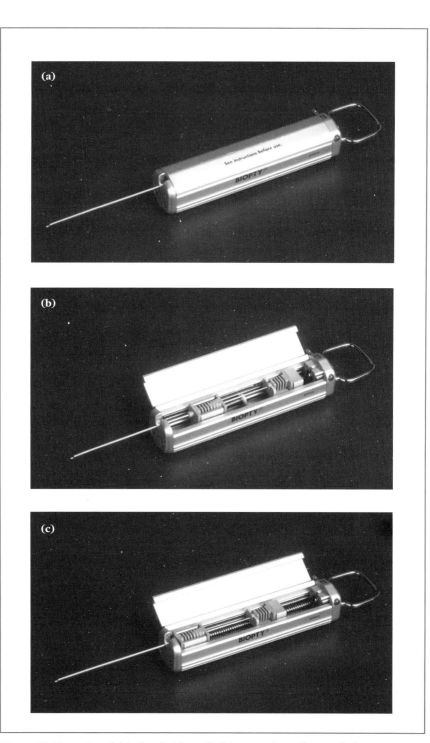

Figure 18. *Biopty Gun. (a) is closed with needle (b) open with needle in cocked position (c) is open with needle in fired position.*

The ultrasound equipment now available is relatively inexpensive and all the instruments have probes that can be programed to guide a biopsy needle to the site of interest. The use of a spring-loaded 'Biopty gun' using an 18 gauge needle enables either transperineal or transrectal ultrasound guided biopsies of suspicious areas to be taken. Prophylactic antibiotic cover for 5 days with a quinalone and metronidazole is obligatory, but anesthesia is not required for this procedure. Multiple biopsies can be performed to sample suspected prostate tumors, even in the absence of obvious lesions on ultrasound. (Figure 18).

What is the diagnostic value of radioisotope bone imaging?

Because prostatic cancer frequently metastasizes to bone, imaging techniques are the next step in staging. The use of radioisotope scintigraphy with bone seeking radioisotopes (99m-Technetium MDP) is an important means of detecting skeletal metastases. Radioisotope scanning is superior to conventional radiology, revealing osseous metastases in approximately 25% of patients with negative findings on X-ray.

A positive scan may precede the appearance of radiologic changes by up to 4 years. It is important in the presence of X-ray positive, isotope-dense areas to exclude false positive scans due to Paget's Disease, degenerative changes, fractures and, rarely, bony infection. The characteristic bony lesions of prostatic carcinoma are osteoblastic. Paget's Disease of the bone produces radiographic areas of increased bone density similar to those of metastatic prostatic cancer. However, in Paget's Disease, the trabecular pattern of the bone is visible, whereas in prostate cancer the trabecular structure is lost, resulting in a smudgy or blurred appearance (Figures 19, 20 and 21).

Since the introduction of PSA for the detection of metastatic disease and the determination of its response to treatment, serial (annual) radionuclide bone scanning is no longer a cost-effective procedure in monitoring the progress of the disease. It can be argued that for newly diagnosed patients with no skeletal symptoms and a PSA < 10 ng/ml, bone scans provide no additional information and if eliminated from the management of such patients, might lead to considerable economic saving to the healthcare system.

Prostate Cancer

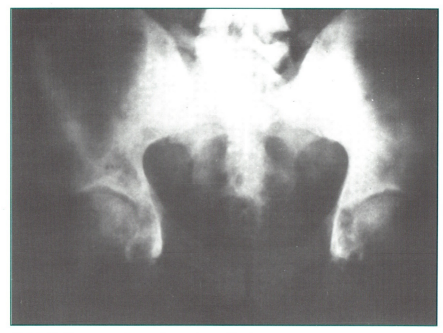

Figure 19. *X-ray, appearances of prostatic osteoblastic metastases.*

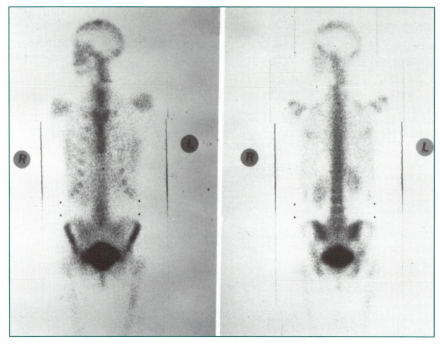

Figure 20. *Normal bone scan.*

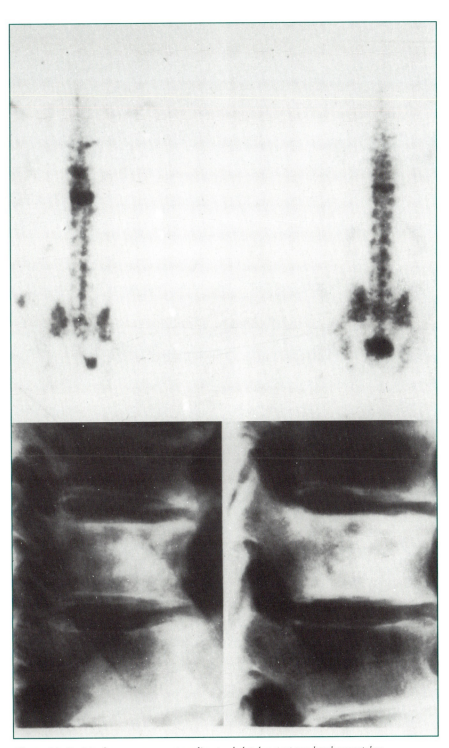

Figure 21. *Positive bone scan corresponding to skeletal metastases lumbar vertebra.*

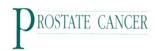
Prostate Cancer

In one study of over 2000 men with newly diagnosed and untreated prostate cancer, 852 had a serum PSA concentration of < 20 ng/ml at the time of presentation. Of these patients, seven (0.8%) had positive bone scans and five of the seven had significant skeletal symptoms. Four of the seven patients had a positive bone scan with a PSA value between 10 and 20 ng/ml, and three had a positive bone scan with a PSA of < 10 ng/ml. However, only one of the three patients with a PSA of < 10 ng/ml and a positive bone scan did not have skeletal symptoms.

Thus, only one of 2000 patients would not have been detected without a bone scan because he was asymptomatic and had a PSA <10 ng/ml (Oesterling, 1993). Clearly, PSA qualifies as an excellent predictor of bone metastases at a cut-off of 10 ng/ml.

Can the bone scan, therefore, be dispensed with in favor of PSA?

Not yet. The bone scan still has important advantages in the staging of prostate cancer. An unequivocally raised PSA may be indicative of metastatic disease, but the bone scan will give a clearer definition of the site and volume of the disease; an important consideration in assessing prognosis. Low-volume disease appears to have a more favorable response to combined hormone ablation.

There is also some evidence that in patients with metastases confined to the axial skeleton, the prognosis is better than when the ribs, lung, ischium and femora are affected. PSA could not provide this information.

Furthermore, with some very poorly differentiated tumors, PSA may be weakly expressed and therefore unrepresentative of widespread bony metastases.

A bone scan also provides an indirect index of renal function and is a prerequisite in the staging of patients suitable for curative radical prostatectomy. My personal preference is for a baseline bone scan, but I no longer use sequential scans to monitor the course of the disease.

What is the role of imaging of the regional lymph nodes in the management of prostate cancer?

When the bone scan and skeletal survey are negative and the cancer is confined to the prostate, imaging of the regional lymph nodes prior to surgery is indicated in a patient suitable for radical prostatectomy or radiotherapy. The primary area of node involvement is a triangle outlined by the external iliac vessels laterally, the hypogastric vasculature medially and the pelvic floor inferiorly.

Some clinicians prefer to perform a laparoscopic staging lymphadenectomy in which all the lymphatic tissue in this area and around the obturator nerve is removed and examined histologically. A computed tomography (CT) scan of the pelvis and abdomen, or a magnetic resonance imaging (MRI) scan of the area can be used to detect node involvement prior to surgery or radiotherapy.

Unfortunately, the accuracy of these investigations is limited and in a small percentage of patients false-negative scans result in the disease being understaged.

What biochemical markers are associated with prostate cancer?

Prostatic acid phosphatase (PAP), the classical and time-honoured serum marker for prostate cancer, has now been superseded by prostate specific antigen (PSA). Many clinicians continue to use, and laboratories to report, both assays, but which one should be done, when, and how often is debatable.

However, there is little doubt that PSA is more sensitive than PAP and it seems to have entered public awareness to an extent that the earlier marker never did.

What is the role of prostatic acid phosphatase?

PAP was the first ever described tumor marker when, in 1938, Gutman and Gutman first recognized the presence of an acid phosphatase in the serum of patients with metastasizing carcinoma of the prostate. The acid phosphatases are a group of phosphohydralases which hydrolyse phosphoric monoesters in an acidic medium. The precise role of acid phosphatases in prostatic epithelium is not known; however, in prostatic fluid they are concerned with the metabolic activity of spermatozoa by catalyzing the transfer of phosphates.

Prostate Cancer

In normal prostate epithelium, there is an orderly process of secretory product synthesis, but in both BPH and prostate cancer there is a decrease in the amount of PAP secreted per cell. The elevations of PAP seen in prostate carcinoma occur because of the overall increase in cell mass, an actual increase in tumor mass, loss of ductal connections, tissue necrosis and neo-vascularization, with subsequent leakage of the enzyme into the circulation. Regional lymphatic spread and distant metastases may establish independent sites of enzyme-secreting tumor.

How is prostatic acid phosphatase measured?

Enzymatic measurement of serum PAP is performed using thymolphthalein monophosphate as the substrate, and L-tartrate inhibition to specifically identify the PAP fraction. Various isoenzymes of serum acid phosphatase have been identified and classified as tartrate-sensitive (the prostate fraction) or tartrate-resistant (the non-prostate fraction).

The tartrate-sensitive fraction, which is supposedly specific for the prostatic fraction of total acid phosphatase, is also found in leukocytes, platelets and other tissues. Normally, the prostatic fraction constitutes only 10–25% of the total serum acid phosphatase found in males, while the platelet fraction constitutes the majority of the remaining fraction.

In 1974, Cooper and Foti described a method of measuring PAP by radioimmunoassay. The technique depends on the specific immunogenicity of the marker and is reportedly independent of other variables affecting enzymatic determinations, such as pH, temperature, and acid phosphatase production from non-prostate cells. However, early reports of the superior sensitivity and specificity of the radioimmunoassay method have not been confirmed.

With clinical experience, it soon became apparent that PAP was not sufficiently sensitive to detect early prostatic cancer. The overall sensitivity for all stages of the disease is approximately 50%. In stage C (T3) and D (T4) disease, the diagnosis is evident clinically by rectal examination and TRUS or history; the PAP determination is merely confirmatory and may only be indicative of the extent of the disease.

Even among patients with advanced metastatic disease, the PAP may be normal in up to 20% of cases. In several studies, the PAP sensitivity for

Stage C and D disease varied from 24% to 92% (cumulative sensitivity for Stage C = 47%; Stage D = 78%). As a marker for early disease, it is far less sensitive (cumulative sensitivity for stage A = 16%; stage B 42%) (Pappas and Gadsden 1984).

Overall, there is no place for PAP in screening the asymptomatic patient and it has lost its role in monitoring the progression or regression of clinical disease, although it is still used by some for this purpose.

Can prostatic acid phosphatase be raised in BPH and in other non-prostate diseases?

Yes, PAP is sometimes elevated in BPH and the values vary according to the assay used. With the enzymatic method it was approximately 6%, with the radioimmunoassay method it was around 10% and with the enzyme linked immunosorbent assay it was 30%. The reasons for the raised PAP in benign disease are: prostatic manipulation during rectal examination, cytolysis of acinar cells, prostatic infarcts and cellular hyperplasia with a concomitant overall increase in enzyme-secreting cells.

It is interesting that PAP elevation occurs in 8% (33/406) of non-prostatic malignancies which tend to be of the 'secretory' type. Elevations have been reported with lymphoma, oat cell carcinoma, carcinoid, renal cell carcinoma adenocarcinoma of lung, breast and pancreas, bladder cancer and multiple myeloma. It is possible that these tumors express one of several substances that have some immunologically similar epitopes as PAP.

What exactly is prostatic specific antigen?

Prostatic specific antigen (PSA) was initially discovered in seminal plasma by Hara et al., in Japan in 1971. Two years later, Li and Beling were able to isolate and characterize PSA as a low molecular weight protein 31,000 daltons, with a slow β-mobility on electrophoresis and a high diffusion rate in agar medium.

In 1979, Wang et al., isolated an antigen from prostatic tissue, purified it and demonstrated its specificity with prostatic tissue. Subsequently, Wang et al demonstrated that PSA found in seminal plasma is immunologically identical and biochemically similar to the antigen that they had isolated from the prostate gland.

Prostate Cancer

Biochemically, PSA is now known to be a single chain glycoprotein that contains 93% amino acids and 7% carbohydrate. It is a monomer with 240-amino acid residues and four carbohydrate side chains. With gel filtration and gel electrophoresis it was found to have a molecular weight of 34,000 daltons.

Functionally, PSA is a kallikrein-like, serine protease that is produced exclusively by the epithelial cells lining the acini and ducts of the prostate gland. Its function is to liquefy the seminal coagulum in the ejaculate. Normally, PSA is secreted into the lumina of the prostatic acini and is present in the seminal plasma in high concentrations. The concentration of PSA in semen ranges from 0.24 to 5.5 mg/ml with a mean of 1.92 mg/ml (Sensabaugh, 1978).

What is the normal range for PSA in serum, and how is it measured?

The most widely used method and the standard reference for the measurement of PSA in the serum has been determined using a solid-phase, two-site immunoradiometric assay that uses two murine monoclonal antibodies for separate epitopes on the PSA molecule (TANDEM - R PSA assay Hybritech. Inc). More than 95% of all commercial and research laboratories use this assay.

The values in all men under 40 years of age, 97% of men 40 or over, and all women of any age were less than or equal to 4.0 ng/ml. In 3% of men 40 or older, serum PSA was greater than 4.0 ng/ml, but not more than 10.0 ng/ml. Consequently, 4.0 ng/ml was selected as the appropriate cut-off concentration to differentiate normal from elevated PSA levels (Myrtle et al.,1986).

Using the mean value plus three standard deviations, investigators at the Johns Hopkins Hospital calculated the upper limit of normal to be 2.0 ng/ml for men less than 40 years old and 2.8 ng/ml for men 40 years or older without prostatic disease (Rock et al., 1987).

As PSA is organ-specific, it is produced by normal, hyperplastic and cancerous prostatic tissue. Concentrations of PSA per gram of tissue do not differ significantly among the three types of prostatic tissue and the marker can be detected in the serum of young men with normal prostates, older men with BPH, and men with localized or metastatic prostatic cancer.

Since BPH and prostate cancer occur in men in the same age range, it is important to understand the relationship between PSA levels and malignant or benign prostatic disease if PSA is to be useful as a tumor marker for prostate cancer.

Stamey et al., (1987) found that 86% of 73 men with BPH had an elevated serum PSA; the preoperative levels ranging from 0.3 to 37 ng/ml, with a mean of 7.9 ng/ml. After a TUR of the prostate, the mean value decreased to 1.3 ng/ml (range 0.1 to 6.7 ng/ml). Based on these findings, the investigators concluded that benign hyperplastic tissue elevated serum PSA level at a rate of 0.3 ng/ml/gm of BPH tissue. However, such a consistent relationship between the amount of BPH and the serum PSA has not been observed by others.

Since only the glandular component produces PSA, the influence of BPH tissue with its morphological heterogeneity is bound to vary and it seems unlikely that a series of normal ranges for a given prostate size could be established. Nevertheless, patients with large benign glands may have PSA levels > 4.0 ng/ml, and approximately 20% of patients with BPH will have PSA levels > 10 ng/ml. A PSA value greater than 4 ng/ml tends to arouse suspicion and is an indication for further evaluation.

There have been attempts to quantify the relationship between gland size and PSA by dividing the concentration in PSA level in ng/ml by the volume of the prostate as determined by ultrasound. The parameter produced is defined as *PSA density*. In a study by Benson et al., (1992) the mean PSA densities for patients with cancer and BPH were 0.581 and 0.044, respectively. Only two cancer patients had a density of 0.05 or less, and no BPH patient had a density higher than 0.117.

Benson et al., used their PSA density calculation in a well characterized population of 533 men, allowing the production of predictive nomograms, giving a PSA density defined cancer risk from 3% to 100%.

Using 'the rate of change in serum PSA' otherwise defined as the *PSA velocity* is said to increase the specificity for distinguishing prostate cancer from BPH. One such study demonstrated an improvement in specificity from 60% to 90% when velocity was considered versus a simple cut-off of

PROSTATE CANCER

4 ng/ml (Carter et al, 1992). Thus, a change from 1.8 ng/ml to 2.9 ng/ml over the course of a year would be significant and might lead to the early detection of a cancer, even though the PSA value remained within the normal range.

How useful is PSA as a tumor marker?

An ideal tumor marker is expressed only by cancer cells and can be detected with reliability at the time the tumor achieves biologic importance. The perfect tumor marker for prostate cancer has not yet been discovered. PSA is not a prostate cancer-specific marker; it is prostate tissue-specific and consequently, other benign conditions of the prostate can influence its serum concentration. Nevertheless, there is a general agreement that serum PSA is a useful and reliable tool in:

- the diagnosis and staging of prostate cancer
- monitoring the response to therapy
- signaling disease progression and establishing a prognosis.

The concentration of serum PSA was found to be > 4 ng/ml (elevated) in 81% of 553 prostate cancer patients; in 46% of these it was greater than 40 ng/ml (Myrtle et al., 1986). The percentage of patients with concentrations of PSA above 4 ng/ml increased progressively through stages A, B, C & D.

In another study, of 378 patients with prostate cancer, the PSA was elevated in 122/127 patients with newly diagnosed untreated prostate cancer, including 7/12 patients with unsuspected early disease, and in all 115 with advanced disease (Stamey et al., 1987).

What is the value of PSA in monitoring a man with metastatic prostatic cancer?

PSA has been found to be raised in about 95–100% of patients with advanced prostate cancer. Several studies have shown that the level falls precipitously with the commencement of first-line anti-androgen therapy and remains low until there is progression of the disease. Patients in whom the PSA level decreases to the normal range (< 2.5 ng/ml) or becomes undetectable by six months after receiving anti-androgen therapy, enjoy a prolonged response to hormonal treatment (Stamey et al., 1989).

PSA concentrations after anti-androgen treatment are inversely proportional to survival time; lower PSA levels correspond with longer survival times, whereas higher concentrations correspond with a shorter survival time.

A fall of serum PSA to normal and/or a drop of 90–95% has important prognostic consequences; those patients who show a profound decline in PSA of 90–95% of the pre-treatment level have a much longer progression-free interval than those who do not.

Prostate Cancer

CHAPTER 3
PATHOLOGY

What factors determine the biologic behavior of prostate cancer?

Perhaps the most important determinant of whether prostate cancer remains innocent and localized or spreads and kills is the biologic behavior of the tumor, which, to some extent, is reflected in its pathologic characteristics.

In order to understand the pathology of prostate cancer, it is necessary to know something of the anatomy of the prostate gland. Our current concept of the anatomy of the prostate is based on the work of McNeil (1984).

Prostate anatomy

The normal prostate gland is a pear-shaped structure, flattened in its antero-posterior dimension with its narrow tapering end, the apex, directed distally, and its broad end, the base, abutting the bladder and seminal vesicles. Its main ducts radiate predominantly laterally from the urethra into the coronal plane, with smaller branches directed posteriorly and to a lesser degree anteriorly. The urethra traverses the prostate eccentrically and most of the tissue anterior to a coronal plane along the long axis of the urethra consists of a thick fibro-muscular stroma.

The bulk of the functional glandular and supporting stromal elements of the prostate gland lie lateral and posterior to the urethra. Thus, the urethra is a key anatomic reference point for study of the glandular tissue. In a sagittal plane (Figure 22), the most important feature of the urethra is an angulation of about 20–30° in its line of axis at about the mid-point of its intraprostatic course.

The base of the verumontanum rests against the posterior wall at the point of angulation. The ejaculatory ducts and the ducts of about 95% of the prostatic glandular tissue enter the urethra in the distal half of the prostatic urethra on either side of the verumontanum.

PROSTATE CANCER

In a coronal section of the gland, two anatomically and histologically separate zones of prostatic glandular tissue can be identified (Figure 23). These have been named the central and the peripheral zones.

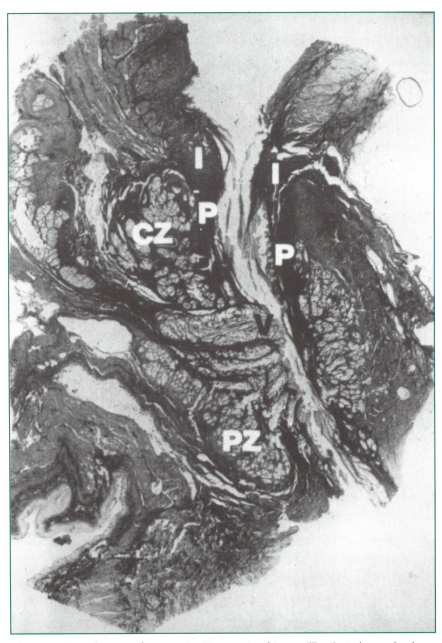

Figure 22. *Sagittal section of prostate: P = Preprostatic sphincter, CZ = Central zone glands, PZ = Peripheral zone glands, V = Verumontanum 20 - 30° angulation of prostate urethra.*

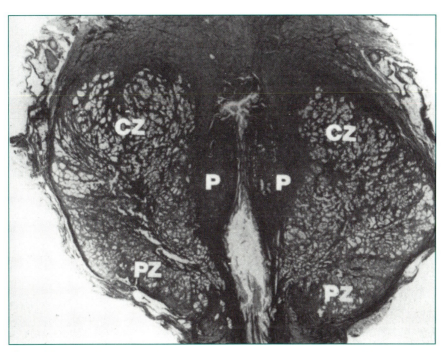

Figure 23. *Coronal section: P = Preprostatic sphincter, CZ = Central zone glands, PZ = Peripheral zone glands.*

The peripheral zone (Figure 24) comprises approximately 75% of the glandular tissue of the prostate. Microscopically, the architecture of the peripheral zone consists of small, simple, round to oval, acinar structures surrounded by a stroma of loosely arranged and randomly interwoven muscle bundles.

The ducts are long and narrow and open into the urethra either at a right angle or with their ostia directed cranially towards the bladder. The ducts and acini are lined by simple columnar epithelium composed of clear cells with basally placed small dark nuclei.

The central zone of the prostate gland (Figure 24) is the wedge of tissue seen in the coronal plane enclosed by the peripheral zone. The ducts and acini of the central zone are much larger than in the peripheral zone and are of irregular outline. The lining epithelium is stratified pseudoepithelium with large pale nuclei lying at different levels in columnar cells having a granular, opaque cytoplasm.

The muscular stroma is much more compact than that of peripheral zone. The ducts of the glands are directed downwards and medially, opening into the urethra in a line parallel with the ejaculatory ducts with which the central zone is intimately related.

Prostate Cancer

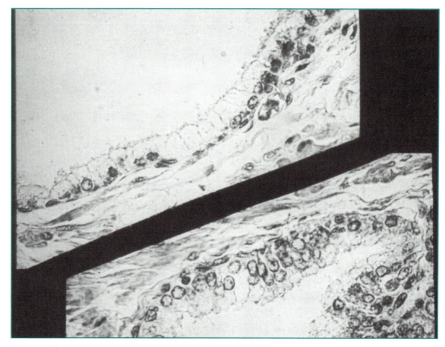

Figure 24. *Histology of prostate. Peripheral zone (above). Central zone (below).*

A double lateral line of peripheral zone ducts continues into the proximal urethral segment, where it gives rise to the remaining 5% of the prostatic glandular tissue which is located in the preprostatic region, the transitional zone.

Although the duct-acinar system here is identical to that of the peripheral zone, there are several reasons to consider this a separate region of glandular tissue. Firstly, the preprostatic gland mass is anatomically displaced anteriorly from the coronal plane of greatest extent of the peripheral zone.

Secondly, there is an abrupt reduction by an order of magnitude in size and degree of development of the duct system from the peripheral zone to the preprostatic region.

Thirdly, the stroma here is different from that of the peripheral zone. Finally, it is within this tissue that BPH (benign prostatic hyperplasia) exclusively arises.

What is the clinical importance of the zonal sub-divisions?

The central zone glands are immune to disease. Carcinoma and prostatitis predominantly arise in the peripheral zone. Tumors tend to arise in two locations in the prostate: the peripheral zone, which renders them more readily palpable on rectal examination; and the transitional zone, where they would be included in the tissue removed on transurethral resection.

Peripheral zone tumors grow outwards through the capsule, spreading along the perineural spaces of the nerves that penetrate the prostate capsule at the upper outer corners at the base of the prostate (where invasion of the seminal vesicles and bladder neck is frequent) and at the apex of the gland. Direct backward spread of the tumor is said to be prevented by the strong layers of Denonvillier's fascia. Thus, invasion of the rectum is extremely rare; however, when it does occur, the rectum may be encircled by tumor, or the tumor may bulge into the rectal lumen causing obstruction; rarely, it may ulcerate into the anterior rectal wall.

Lymphatic and hematological spread results in metastases to the pelvic and para-aortic lymph nodes and, overwhelmingly, to the bones, most commonly the lumbar spine, femora and pelvis. Spinal involvement frequently extends into the epidural space causing cord compression with all its neurologic sequelae, from sensory loss and motor weakness to paralysis. Spread to the lungs and liver is less commonly seen with prostate cancer.

What is the role of the pathologist in the management of prostatic cancer?

The criteria for the pathologic diagnosis of prostatic cancer are disturbance of the normal architecture, invasion, and anaplasia (Mostofi et al., 1992). The extent to which these features are present denotes the biologic behavior of the tumor, helps the clinician plan a treatment strategy and, finally, determines the outcome.

What are the histological features of prostate cancer?

In the normal prostate, the glands radiating from the urethra and the acini have a characteristic convoluted appearance. These features are lost in prostate cancer.

Disturbances are manifested as a haphazard distribution of glands, small and large acini closely packed together, large acini without convolutions, fused glands, glands in glands, rare glands or columns and cords or solid sheets. In cancer, instead of a double layer of cells lining the acini (as seen in BPH) there may be a single layer of cells or piling up of cells with many cancers showing more than one growth pattern (see the Gleason System, Figures 7-12).

Invasion

Invasion is an important criterion for diagnosis. The acini of normal and hyperplastic glands are surrounded by a delicate basement membrane which can be demonstrated by laminin stains. There is often an elastic tissue network demonstrable by electron microscopy surrounding the acini and the whole is invested by smooth muscle strands.

Malignant acini do not have this orderly connective tissue framework. The normal arrangement of elastic tissue is not seen in carcinomatous areas. However, this may not be apparent in hematoxylin and eosin stains. Although the earliest sign of invasion is the absence of a basal cell layer, this is not always reliable because some hyperplastic acini lack a basal cell layer. Breakthrough of the basement membrane is an early indication of stromal invasion.

Stromal invasion can be recognized by the loss of acinar-stromal interaction, as evidenced by the distribution of acini, without regard to the regular whorls of smooth muscle fibres, irregularity of the shape of acini, pointed edges of acini and the presence of outgrowths of individual or groups of neoplastic cells near acini or scattered in the stroma.

Perineural invasion has been seen as indisputable evidence of invasion. When adequate tissue is available, perineural invasion has been found in more than 90% of cases (Mostofi et al., 1992). Vascular and lymphatic invasion is often difficult to recognize in needle biopsy or TUR specimens. This is, in part, the result of diathermy cauterization and squeeze effect. By contrast with capillaries, which are in an intimate relationship with acini, lymphatics are only present in the stroma.

It has been shown that intraprostatic perineural invasion has no clinical significance. However, it may proceed to perineural invasion in the periprostatic tissue and this should be looked for as a staging criterion in radical prostatectomy specimens. In needle biopsy specimens, invasion of periprostatic tissue can be recognized by the presence of neoplastic acini in a fibroadipose stroma and in ganglion cells. It is necessary to report the presence of a tumor outside the prostate as it affects the clinical staging of the tumor and the management of the patient. Special cytokeritin stains may be able to identify isolated malignant cells in the periprostatic tissues.

Nuclear anaplasia

The third and most important criterion in the diagnosis of prostate cancer is nuclear aplasia. In benign prostatic epithelium, the nuclei are small, round and vesicular and may have one delicate nucleolus. In cancer, the nuclei are usually large, and there are variable degrees of differences in shape, size and staining. The chromatin is condensed at the periphery and there is vacuolization of the nuclei.

The most important criterion for diagnosis of nuclear aplasia is the presence of a large nucleolus in the secretory cells. More than one nucleolus may be present and the nucleoli may be centrally or peripherally placed. It should be emphasized that the presence of nucleoli per se is not diagnostic of cancer, because small nuclei are often visible in secretory and basal cells. However, in many well differentiated prostate cancers the presence of large nucleoli is diagnostic.

Prostate Cancer

CHAPTER FOUR

THE CLINICAL MANAGEMENT OF PROSTATE CANCER

When all the clinical, laboratory and radiologic evidence is made available, it transpires that 70–80% of patients with prostate cancer have either locally advanced or metastatic disease (T3, T4, M1 or D2). The treatment for these patients is palliative with some form of hormonal manipulation. The management of patients with localized early prostate cancer is more problematic and controversial, particularly in the younger age group.

How should patients with early stage (stage T1, T2, stage A and B) localized disease be managed?

Locally confined prostate cancer is diagnosed in two ways. Carcinoma detected by chance in the prostate resected or enucleated for clinically benign disease is termed 'incidental prostatic cancer'. It accounts for 4–30% of all cancers of the prostate and its likelihood depends upon the patient's age and the methods of histologic diagnosis.

A much smaller percentage of patients with stage T2 or B, localized disease are diagnosed as a result of rectal examination and biopsy of a suspicious nodule or induration of a prostate lobe. The introduction of screening programs using a combination of DRE, PSA and TRUS will undoubtedly increase the diagnostic yield of these tumors.

The biologic behavior of incidental carcinoma is not uniform, but correlates with the tumor volume and grading. Jewett divided these tumors into A1 and A2.

♦ A1 tumors are well differentiated, focal lesions occupying < 10% of the resected material or < 3 chips. (The extent of focal involvement has varied from < 5% to < 25% with different authors.)
♦ A2 tumors show diffuse > 10 – > 25% or > 3 chips of tissue involvement, with a moderately or poorly differentiated tumor.

PROSTATE CANCER

According to the TNM staging, these are categorized as T1a (< 5% of tissue resected), or T1b (> 5% of resected tissue involved).

Clinical studies have shown that A1 (T1a), well differentiated tumors have a very good prognosis and seldom progress. Patients with A1 disease have a survival which corresponds to the life-expectancy of normal controls matched for age (Figure 25).

Patients with multifocal, poorly differentiated A2 (T1b) tumors usually have a bad prognosis due to early progression and a high incidence of lymph node involvement. In terms of malignancy, an A2 tumor is the same as a palpable B2 tumor. Indeed, patients with A2 G3 tumor had a survival as low as those with a C lesion (Figure 26).

The two most important factors in the prognosis of incidental carcinoma are the volume of the disease and the grade of the tumor. There is general agreement that small volume, incidental prostate carcinoma (A1 [T1a] disease), does not require treatment, but only close observation. Such patients are more likely to die with, not from, their cancers.

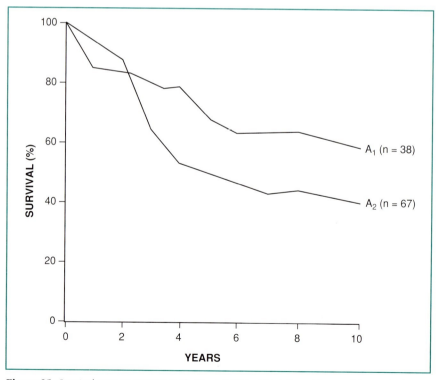

Figure 25. *Survival rates in patients with A1 and A2 incidental carcinoma of the prostate.*

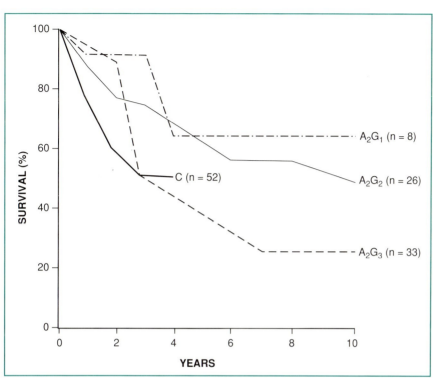

Figure 26. *Survival rates in patients with stage A2 incidental prostate cancer classified according to histological grade.*

What are the treatment options for patients with large volume, moderately or poorly differentiated localized carcinoma?

Firstly, a clearer definition is required for the volume of the disease. Is it to be defined as 5% or 10%, or in terms of the number of chips involved? In most series, a second look TUR has resulted in up-staging of the tumor, indicating that roughly 10% of tumors are understaged on the first TUR.

The second most important consideration is the age of the patient and his life expectancy. In a patient with a life expectancy of 10+ years with negative regional lymph nodes and who is willing to undergo aggressive therapy, radical nerve-sparing prostatectomy is the treatment of choice.

In those who do not consent to surgery, or are unfit for it, radiation therapy is a valid option. There is a higher rate of complications with radiotherapy carried out after a TUR.

Prostate Cancer

The more aggressive and radical approach to localized prostate cancer adopted within recent years has resulted in a widely contested debate about the need for screening the male population at risk of prostate cancer. It seems unlikely to be resolved until there is proof that radical ablative surgery cures patients with localized A2, B or T1b, T2, disease who would otherwise die from their disease if left untreated. The case for screening for prostatic cancer will be discussed later.

What is the treatment for advanced (stage C [T3] and D [T4], M1) prostate cancer?

In 1941, Huggins et al., in a seminal publication, described the favorable effect of orchidectomy and estrogen administration on the progress of metastatic prostate cancer and demonstrated conclusively, for the first time, the responsiveness of prostatic cancer to androgen deprivation. Although the mechanism of endocrine dependence of prostate cancer was not fully understood at the time, a new era had begun in the management of patients with prostate cancer (Figure 27).

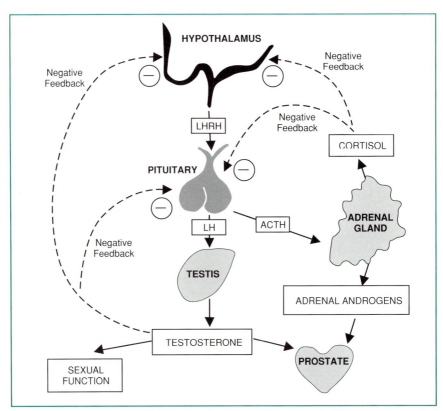

Figure 27. *Endocrine control of testicular function.*

Since that time, endocrine manipulation by androgen blockade has been the mainstay of the management of metastatic prostatic cancer. It is achieved by either surgical castration or drug therapy (medical castration) using anti-androgens, LH-RH analogs, or estrogens.

Most men (approximately 70-80%) surgically or chemically castrated have an initial, often instant and dramatically beneficial response to androgen withdrawal therapy.

However, although this initial response is of considerable palliative value, nearly all treated patients will eventually relapse to an androgen-insensitive state and succumb to progression of the disease, unless they die of intercurrent disease first.

How effective is orchidectomy in the management of metastatic prostate cancer?

Bilateral orchidectomy, either total or subcapsular, continues to be the 'gold standard' of hormonal therapy for metastatic prostatic carcinoma. It has the desired effect of rapidly reducing circulating androgen to < 50 ng/100 ml (10% of normal values). The hormone-responsive prostatic cancer will shrink and the patient will be relieved of his symptoms of bone pain from metastases. A favorable response can be expected in about 70-80% of patients treated with orchidectomy.

The advantages of orchidectomy over forms of medical castration are the lack of feminizing side-effects, gastro-intestinal disorders, and hepatic and cardiovascular complications, and the freedom from the necessity to take regular medication. The latter factor is particularly useful in some frail and forgetful old men.

Impotence is not an inevitable consequence of orchidectomy, but is more than likely to ensue. After castration, there is a rise in serum LH-RH and luteinizing hormone (LH) levels, the effects of which are loss of libido and hot flushes.

Does orchidectomy provide adequate endocrine control?

There is little evidence that orchidectomy is clinically less effective than other forms of monotherapy. However, there is a need to address the question of whether orchidectomy is enough to deprive the tumor of all its androgen requirement.

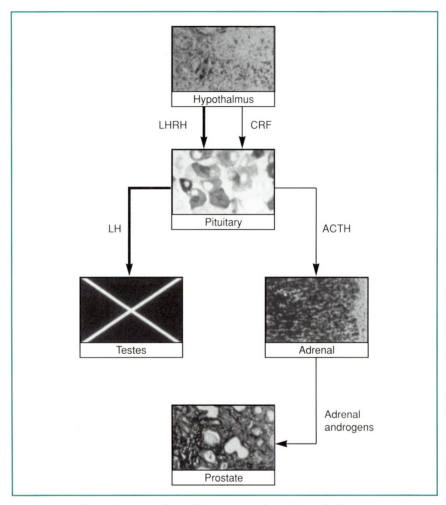

Figure 28. *Androgen deprivation by orchidectomy or subcapsular orchidectomy.*

There is evidence that deprivation of testicular androgen results in atrophy of the normal prostate, and adrenal androgens alone do not seem to be capable of maintaining growth and function of the human prostate (Oesterling et al., 1986). (Figure 28). But is this also true of the malignant prostate?

Geller et al., (1978), showed that after orchidectomy in patients with prostate cancer, tissue levels of dihydrotestosterone (DHT) in the prostate were reduced by only 60–70%. The residue must, therefore, be derived from adrenal androgen which, clearly, makes a sizeable contribution to androgen metabolism within the prostate gland (Figure 29).

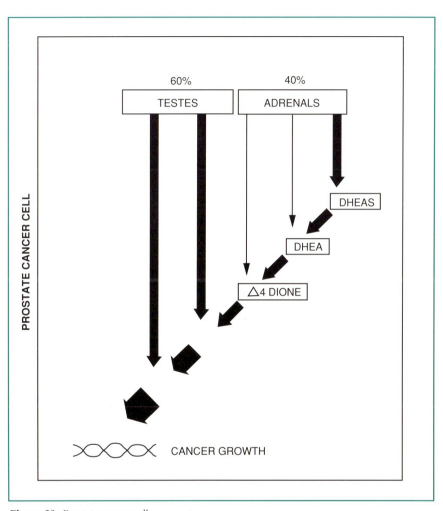

Figure 29. *Prostate cancer cell.*

The question of whether or not the amounts of androgen found in the prostate after castration maintain growth of the tumor and subsequently lead to clinically detectable differences in response, progression and death has not been satisfactorily answered. The question of how much androgen prostate cancer requires to grow also awaits an answer.

It must also be borne in mind that for some men, castration is an unacceptable assault on their manhood, and that such sentiments must be respected.

Prostate Cancer

What is the place of estrogens in the treatment of prostate cancer, and how do they work?

Estrogens are considered to produce their main effects indirectly by suppressing the secretion of LH-RH from the hypothalamus, thereby inhibiting the release of LH from the pituitary. Without this suppression, LH-RH would act on the pituitary to stimulate the secretion of LH, which acts on the Leydig cells of the testes to produce testosterone (Figure 30).

Direct effects of estrogens on the testes may also contribute to depressed androgen synthesis. This has been demonstrated in experiments where estradiol-17β was shown to suppress testosterone levels in gonadotrophin

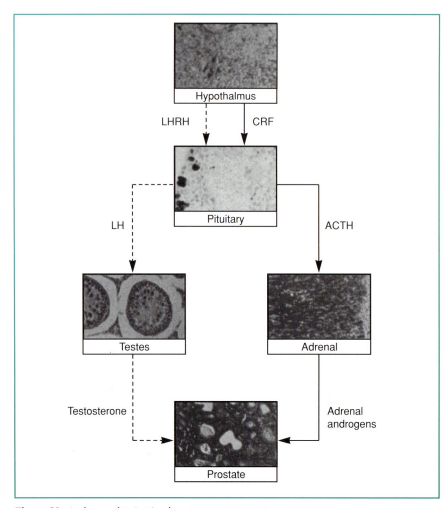

Figure 30. *Androgen deprivation by estrogens or progestogens.*

substituted hypophysectomized rats (Melner and Abney, 1980), and in vitro studies in which estradiol induced a dose-dependent inhibition of gonadotrophin-stimulated testosterone release from human testicular slices, suggesting a direct inhibitory effect on human Leydig cells (Daehlin et al., 1985).

In rats, Leydig cells contain estrogen receptors. Whether these receptors participate in the physiologic regulation of Leydig cell function is controversial. In the human testis, Murphy et al., (1980), demonstrated the presence of low levels of specific nuclear E-2 binding.

Although the estrogenic effect on the prostate is principally via the testis, there is some evidence that estrogens also have a direct effect on the prostate, resulting in inhibition of 5α reductase (Shimazaki et al., 1971; Kadohama et al., 1977), inhibition of DNA- polymerase (Harper et al., 1970) and the existence of estrogen receptors (Bashirelahi et al., 1979; Dahlberg et al., 1980).

Do estrogens have a direct effect on prostate carcinoma cells?

The growth of the Dunning rat adenocarcinoma was shown to be inhibited by the estrogens diethystilboestrol (DES) (Shessel et al., 1980) and estramustine phosphate, Estracyt (Muntzing et al., 1977). Human prostatic carcinomas certainly contain estrogen receptors (Sidh et al., 1979), but there is no clear evidence that estrogens act directly on prostatic carcinoma cells. It was thought that very large doses of estrogen might have a tumoricidal action. The idea was supported by the evidence that increasing the dose of DES from a few milligrams to several hundred milligrams per day increased clinical improvement and further decreased PAP and bone pain (Colapinto and Aberhart, 1961; Trafford, 1965; Rohlf and Flocks, 1969).

DES was the estrogen in most popular use in the early days of hormonal treatment, but several new synthetic estrogenic substances have now been introduced.

In Sweden, estrogens are still an acceptable alternative hormonal therapy for prostate cancer and the drugs commonly used are estramustine phosphate and ethinyl estradiol in combination with polyestradiol phosphate.

PROSTATE CANCER

In one study, 244 men with stage I, II and III prostate cancer were randomized to three groups of treatment:

- polyestradiol phosphate (Estradurin) + ethinyl estradiol
- estramustine phosphate (Estracyt)
- no therapy.

During follow-up for 4.5 years, cardiovascular complications (including ischemic heart disease, cardiac decompensation, cerebral ischemia and venous thromboembolism) were noted in 24 patients in group A, nine in group B, but only one in group C (Lundgren et al., 1986). Similarly, a study by Henrikson and Edhag (1986) found that 25% of patients experienced a serious cardiovascular event necessitating hospitalization within 5 months of starting treatment.

Side-effects of estrogens

Few clinicians now favor the use of estrogens as palliative treatment, due to the high risk of cardiovascular side effects and thromboembolic phenomena. Low-dose stilboestrol (1 mg t.d.s.) may have less associated cardiovascular risk, but even a small dose of estrogen is said to affect platelet aggregability.

Moreover, the side-effects of gynecomastia, breast tenderness, depression, hot flushes, vomiting and nausea associated with estrogen therapy can be very distressing for the patient. Gynecomastia may be prevented by superficial radiation to the breast tissue at a dose of up to 15 Gy before the start of estrogen therapy, and some clinicians advocate the use of 1–3 mg stilboestrol daily, but the question of whether low dose estrogens are preferable to orchidectomy has not been tested by a controlled clinical trial.

The cardiovascular deaths associated with stilboestrol (5 mg/day), first reported in the VACURG (Veterans Administration Cooperative Urological Research Group) study published in 1967, offset the reduced cancer mortality from treatment and highlighted the dangers of estrogen therapy. 'What estrogen treatment wins from cancer, it more than loses to other causes of death' was the salutary message from the study.

Cardiovascular complications are related to the dose of estrogen and to previous cardiovascular morbidity; 85% appear within the first year after the start of treatment. Studies comparing cholesterol ester metabolism in patients treated with orchidectomy, estrogens or cyproterone have shown increases in high density lipoprotein (HDL) and tryglycerides (TG), while total cholesterol (TC) decreased or was unchanged (Rossner et al., 1985).

Cyproterone acetate lowered total cholesterol, LDL (low density lipoprotein) and HDL concentrations (Wallentin and Varenhorst, 1981). Low dose estrogen and anti-androgens (Cyproterone) produce some effects on lipoprotein metabolism, but these are probably of minor importance for the development of atherosclerotic manifestations (Rossner et al., 1985).

Although no results from a controlled study have been reported, the platelet aggregating effects of estrogens can probably be counteracted by the daily use of aspirin (30mg/day).

Estrogens cause a substantial increase in the secretion of prolactin. A number of studies have shown that prolactin intensifies the action of androgens on RNA synthesis in the prostate. Androgen uptake by the prostate is also facilitated by prolactin. Estrogen therapy marks a reduction of androgen concentrations as does orchidectomy, although the secretion of adrenal androgens (above all androstendione and dihydroepiandrosterone) is unimpaired.

What is the place of anti-androgens in the treatment of prostate cancer?

The only factor that has been established as playing an important role in regulation of normal prostate growth is the androgen receptor, a ligand-dependent transcription factor which, after activation by interaction with testosterone or DHT, is able to regulate the expression of specific target genes.

The androgen receptor is essential for normal prostate development, growth and function. In addition, a functionally active androgen receptor is a prerequisite for the growth of androgen-dependent prostate tumors. The androgen receptor might function in an identical way as part of the molecular processes underlying both normal development and androgen-dependent malignant growth.

The male steroid hormones, testosterone (T) and DHT are the ligands for the androgen receptor. The molecular mechanism of androgen receptor action is summarized in Figure 31. In the prostate, T is metabolised to DHT by the enzyme 5 a reductase. The DHT-androgen-receptor complex is able to activate transcription of the specific target genes, which can include genes essential for prostate function and genes involved in prostate growth and development.

There is now ample evidence, mainly from immunohistochemical studies with monospecific antibodies, that the steroid receptors are located in the nucleus of the cell, in both the absence and the presence of the ligand.

An obvious and rational approach to pharmacologic research in prostate cancer disease was to target the androgen receptor-ligand binding. This resulted in the development of the anti-androgens. Anti-androgens can be sub-divided as follows:

Pure (non-steroidal) anti-androgens
♦ Flutamide
♦ Nilutamide
♦ Casodex.

Steroidal (anti-gonadotropically active) anti-androgens
♦ Cyproterone acetate
♦ Megestrol acetate.

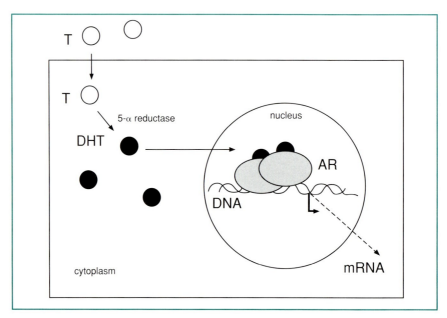

Figure 31. *Schematic diagram of the molecular mechanism of androgen receptor action. T = testosterone, DHT = dihydrotestosterone, AR = androgen receptor.*

The non-steroidal, pure anti-androgens block the function of the androgen receptor without affecting testosterone production, while the steroidal anti-androgens not only block androgen receptor activity, but also inhibit testosterone production (Figure 32).

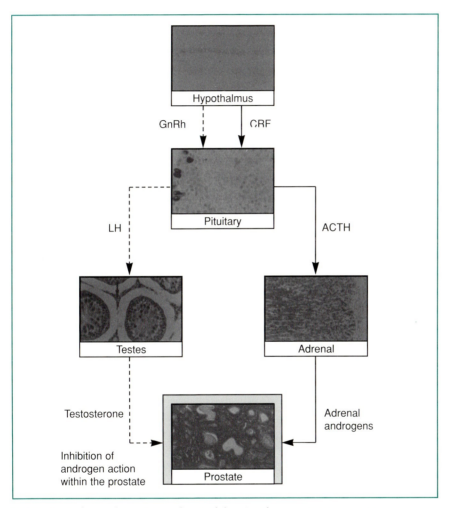

Figure 32. *Androgen deprivation with steroidal anti-androgen cyproterone acetate.*

What is the place of the steroidal anti-androgen, cyproterone acetate as monotherapy in the treatment of advanced prostate cancer?

The hydroxyprogesterone derivative, cyproterone acetate (CPA), was synthesized by Wiechert in 1961 and first used for the treatment of female hirsutism, acne, seborrhea and baldness.

Prostate Cancer

Although there were reports of early clinical trials in the treatment of prostatic carcinoma, its importance and value in this indication was not realized for another 15 years (Scott and Schirmer, 1966; Neumann, 1983).

How does cyproterone acetate act?

CPA is a synthetic 21-carbon steroid that blocks the C21-19 desmolase enzyme and thus inhibits testosterone production by the testes. Although it has a weak progestational effect, it is sufficient to inhibit gonadotrophin secretion and so lower testosterone to castration levels. At the prostatic, intracellular level, it inhibits cytosolic DHT binding and the formation of a nuclear chromatin-DHT-receptor complex without reduction of cytoplasmic androgen up-take and turn-over.

These actions make CPA suitable as first-line hormone treatment as an alternative to orchidectomy and LH-RH analogs. Another effect of its progestational activity is the suppression of hot flushes after orchidectomy.

The difference between the steroidal anti-androgen, cyproterone, and a pure, non-steroidal anti-androgen such as flutamide, is the lack of a progestational effect of the latter, which always causes serum testosterone to rise. The toxic side-effects of the two types of drugs are also different.

Several clinical trials have compared cyproterone with orchidectomy, flutamide, estrogens and LH-RH analogs for androgen deprivation. There appear to be no differences between any of the treatment regimens in terms of time-to-progression or survival.

What are the side-effects of cyproterone acetate?

The incidence of cardiovascular and thromboembolic complications is much less than with estrogens. It should, of course, be avoided in patients with a known cardiovascular risk. Gynecomastia is usually mild and does not necessitate withdrawal of the drug. A significant advantage of CPA is its ability to reduce and suppress the hot flushes that often accompany orchidectomy and LH-RH agonist therapy. Like other forms of androgen deprivation, cyproterone causes impotence and a loss of libido.

Cyproterone acetate is said to be the anti-androgen of choice to be used in combination with LH-RH analogs at the start of treatment to prevent the disease-flare (Figure 33).

Pure anti-androgens are less desirable here, as they stimulate serum testosterone to rise, with largely unknown effects on the cancer process. Testosterone secretion could continue to rise to an extent that it overcomes the blocking effect of anti-androgens on the prostate. The superiority of cyproterone in this respect has been disputed.

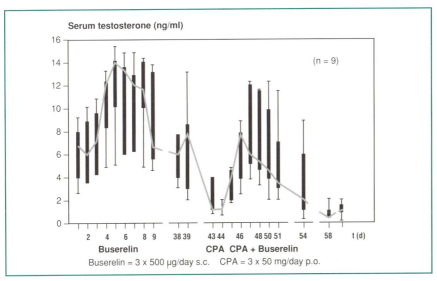

Figure 33. *Inhibitory effect of cyproterone acetate (CPA) on the increase in serum testosterone level during the initial stimulatory phase in men treated with the LH-RH agonist Buserelin.*

What is the rationale for the use of non-steroidal anti-androgens in the management of prostate cancer?

There is now substantial evidence that this group of drugs produce a favorable clinical response in metastatic disease. Flutamide (alpha, alpha, alpha-trifluoro-2-methyl-4-nitro-m-propionotoluidide), a derivative of toluidine has been shown to inhibit nuclear androgen binding in animals, and to be effective against several of the androgens known to be involved in prostate cancer, including testosterone, DHT and androstenedione. Any of these androgens when given to orchidectomized rats causes rapid regrowth of the prostate which may be successfully blocked by flutamide in various doses.

Orally administered, flutamide is converted to hydroxyflutamide which acts as a non-competitive receptor antagonist. It is well absorbed, highly protein bound in vivo, with a half life of about 8–10 hours and is excreted primarily in the urine. Studies have shown that the binding affinity of flutamide for the receptor is significantly less than the affinity of the androgen for the receptor.

What are the results of clinical studies with flutamide?

Flutamide has been used in clinical practice for many years. In patients with metastatic prostate cancer who were previously untreated, the response rate averages about 85%. In comparative studies with stilboestrol there was no statistically significant difference between the two therapies. This indicates that flutamide is probably as effective as either 1 mg or 3 mg of DES, and probably as effective as other hormonal manipulations.

Compared with DES, there is less cardiovascular toxicity. In patients who had previously failed on hormonal therapy the response to flutamide was seen to be about 30% (Stollar and Albert, 1974; Sogani and Whitmore, 1979).

The National Cancer Institute intergroup protocol investigated patients who had been given leuprolide plus placebo and failed. About half of these patients opted to take flutamide, but it did not improve survival. At present, flutamide is not FDA-approved in the United States as monotherapy for metastatic prostatic cancer, but can be used in conjunction with Gn-RH analogs.

One of the significant advantages of treatment with flutamide is the preservation of potency in approximately 75% of patients. Men given flutamide show increased levels of both LH and testosterone. By 12 months, however, the elevated testosterone levels have returned to normal (Lund and Rasmussen, 1988). Flutamide monotherapy should be considered in selected patients with metastatic prostatic cancer wishing to retain their sexual function, provided initial PSA levels do not exceed 120 ng/ml. The patient's testosterone and PSA levels should be closely monitored.

Are there any adverse side-effects of flutamide treatment?

A troublesome problem with flutamide therapy is gynecomastia, which occurs in about 50% of cases. The mechanism is unknown, though it may be related to increases in circulating testosterone, estradiol or estrone. The ratio of estrogen to testosterone is increased by flutamide and can even be boosted with aromatization of testosterone to estrogen. Estrogens may modulate the receptor content of the breast tissue, but flutamide itself has no direct activity on the breast (Benson, 1992).

Diarrhoea occurs in 25% of patients given flutamide, but this is usually manageable and not too bothersome. Hepatotoxicity causing jaundice is an unusual event. Worldwide, in a three year period, there were 88 reports of such events (0.9 events per 1000 patient years) (Benson, 1992), all of which promptly resolved with discontinuation of the drug. Despite this low incidence of hepatotoxicity, liver function tests should be performed at one, three and six months and at six monthly intervals thereafter.

What is the role of LH-RH agonists in the treatment of prostate cancer?

LH-RH is a decapeptide originally described in 1969. Normally, this hormone binds to receptors on the cell surface in the pituitary, and the receptor-hormone complex stimulates production of LH which then passes into the circulation and binds to LH receptors on the surface of the Leydig cells in the testes. The LH-receptor complex is then transported into the nucleus where it activates the cyclic AMP-protein kinase system and induces production of testosterone.

Secretion of LH and follicle-stimulating hormone (FSH) by the pituitary from puberty onwards provides the gonadotrophic stimulation for the development of the testes and androgen-dependent organs in the adult reproductive male.

Physiologic control of LH and FSH secretion by the pituitary requires a pulsatile delivery of low doses of Gn-RH (LH-RH) from the hypothalamus with a relatively constant frequency of 60–120 per minute. If this pattern is significantly altered, either by increasing the dose or the frequency, or by a continuous infusion, inhibition or down-regulation (desensitization) of the pituitary results, and LH and FSH secretion ceases (Figure 34).

The discovery of LH-RH and its mechanism of action seemed to present an opportunity to treat hypogonadism and infertility. Of all the hypothalamic hormones identified thus far, LH-RH has undergone perhaps the most extensive and successful chemical modification and pharmacologic

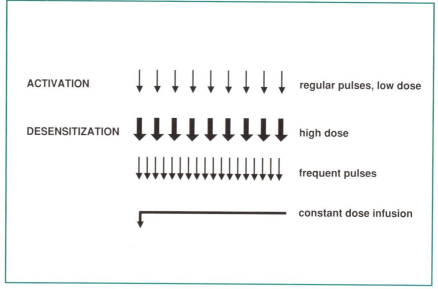

Figure 34. *Densitization of the pituitary.*

development. Approximately 1,600 synthetic analogs of LH-RH have been developed. Substitution of the amino acids at positions 6 or 10 (or both) produced analogs with a biologic activity approximately 30 times greater than natural LH-RH.

Chronic treatment of animals with these compounds produced an array of hormonal and reproductive effects consonant with medical castration.

Redding and Schally (1981), showed that one of these analogs significantly inhibited the growth of prostatic tumors in male rats. The identification and synthesis of these superactive analogs of LH-RH heralded a new treatment modality for hormone-dependent prostatic cancer.

In clinical practice, four have gained worldwide popularity; leuprorelin, goserelin, buserelin and nafarelin (Figure 35). At present, only leuprorelin and goserelin have been approved by the FDA in the United States.

How are LH-RH agonists administered?

These drugs cannot be given orally as they would be destroyed by peptic digestion. At first, they were administered as daily subcutaneous injections (goserelin) or as an intra-nasal spray (buserelin).

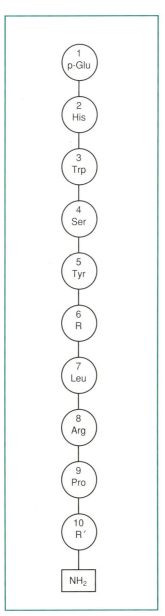

Figure 35. *Amino acid sequences of some GnRH analogs used in prostatic cancer:*
*leuprorelin (**R** = D-leucine; **R'** = ethyllamide); goserelin (**R** = D-serine ter-butyl;*
***R'** = ethylamide); nafarelin (**R** = D-naphthylalanine; **R'** = glycine); GnRH*
*(**R** = **R** = glycine).*

The inconvenience of daily injections and the uncertainty of intra-nasal administration have now been successfully overcome by the introduction of biodegradable depot formulations that ensure better patient compliance and the controlled release of LH-RH analog over a 30-day period. Longer acting depot formulations are in preparation.

What is disease flare?

For the first two weeks after the start of treatment with an LH-RH analog, there is initial stimulation of the pituitary prior to its desensitization which results in a rapid rise in serum testosterone levels. This sudden surge in testosterone production can produce a flare-up of the patient's symptoms with an increase in bone pain within two to three days (Figures 36 and 37).

Treatment with an LH-RH analog is known to have precipitated spinal cord compression resulting in paraplegia and ureteric obstruction in some patients with spinal secondaries and impending ureteric obstruction.

This flare phenomenon occurs in about 4% of patients but can be avoided by concomitant treatment with an anti-androgen started seven to ten days before the first injection of LH-RH (simultaneous administration does not prevent the surge of serum testosterone) and continued for two weeks thereafter. With continued LH-RH treatment, the serum testosterone falls to castration levels and no rise in testosterone levels is seen with subsequent injections.

Prostate Cancer

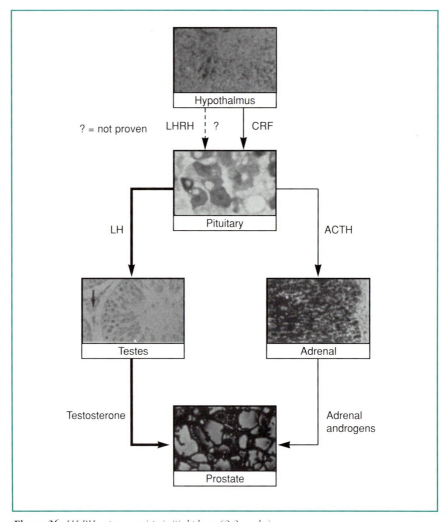

Figure 36. *LH-RH-superagonists-initial phase (2-3 weeks).*

How effective is LH-RH in the treatment of prostate cancer?

Several studies have shown that suppression of gonadal steroidogenesis can be achieved by the sustained administration of long-acting LH-RH analogs. Serum testosterone is reduced to castration levels, there is relief of bone pain and a reduction in PAP and PSA within four weeks of commencing treatment.

Sequential ultrasonography has shown a reduction in the size of the prostate by approximately 50%. Randomized, controlled, clinical trials have shown that LH-RH is as effective as orchidectomy or DES 1 mg t.i.d. in the treatment of metastatic prostate cancer.

A phase III study by the British Prostate Group (Peeling, 1989) comparing goserelin with orchidectomy and DES reported no significant differences in either subjective (goserelin 66% *vs* orchidectomy 75%) or objective (goserelin 71% *vs* orchidectomy 72%) response between treatments, and the mean times to objective response were similar.

The time to progression of the disease (treatment failure) and survival did not differ significantly between the various treatment groups. The median survival periods in the groups were approximately two years (goserelin - 115 weeks; orchidectomy - 104 weeks).

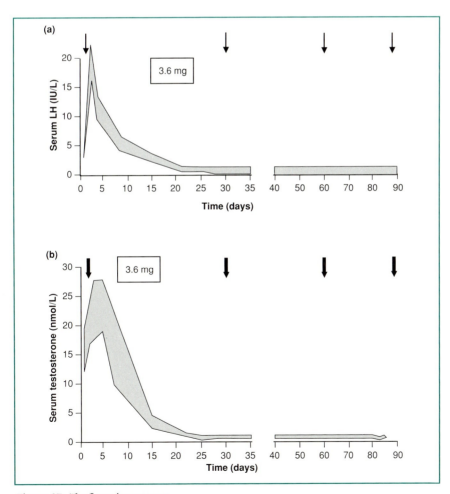

Figure 37. *The flare phenomenon.*

Prostate Cancer

LH-RH analogs appear to be well tolerated; the major side-effect is hot flushes which occur as frequently as with castration and estrogen therapy. The analogs are devoid of the cardiovascular and thromboembolic risks of estrogens.

What is total androgen blockade?

Orchidectomy eliminates testicular androgen and reduces circulating testosterone levels by 90%; the remaining 10% being derived from adrenal sources. After LH-RH treatment, 5% of endogenous testosterone and testosterone-producing capacity of the testicular tissue remains.

Although the serum testosterone concentrations fall to one tenth of normal, the amount of androgen detectable in prostatic cancer tissue may amount to 40–50% of normal, mostly derived from the intra-prostatic metabolism of adrenal androgen (Geller et al., 1984).

Do low remaining levels of androgen compromise the effect of the treatment, and therefore, should they be eliminated as well?

This can be achieved by either blocking the synthesis and/or the release of adrenal and testicular androgen, or by blocking the intracellular biochemical steps which mediate androgen action in target tissues.

Intracellular blockade of androgen can be achieved by inhibiting the binding of DHT to the nuclear membrane receptors, or by inhibition of the 5α reductase which converts testosterone to DHT. The combination of an LH-RH analog with an anti-androgen, or orchidectomy with an anti-androgen, would effectively result in total androgen blockade or, more precisely, combined androgen blockade.

The 5α reductase inhibitor, finasteride, that permits testosterone to be spared but blocks its conversion to the active metabolite, DHT, has not as yet been fully tested in the treatment of prostate cancer.

Is combined androgen blockade more effective than monotherapy?

In 1983, Labrie and his co-workers in Canada treated patients with advanced metastatic prostatic cancer with a combination of the Gn-RH analog, leuprorelin and the pure, non-steroidal, anti-androgen, flutamide. The rationale of this approach was that flutamide would inhibit the intracellular steroid-receptor binding of circulating androgens of adrenal origin which could have a stimulatory effect on the prostate cancer cell after the suppression of testicular androgen by the Gn-RH analog. The investigators reported that this combined androgen blockade led to a dramatic improvement in survival, as well as in time to progression, in patients with stage D2 disease and bony metastases. The authors claimed 90% survival at two years, compared with an otherwise average two-year survival of 40–60%. In addition, they reported that progression of disease at 17 months averaged 26%, compared with 70% in a control group treated with either leuprorelin or DES 3 mg/day alone.

Other investigators have failed to reproduce these spectacular results. Nevertheless, in a large prospective multi-center study of 603 patients in the United States, carried out by the Southwest Oncology Group and sponsored by the National Cancer Institute, a combination of leuprolide with flutamide or placebo produced a statistically significant difference in progression-free survival in favor of the group receiving leuprolide and flutamide.

The median progression-free survival time was 16.5 months for the flutamide group and 13.9 months for the placebo group (Figure 38). The median lengths of survival were 35.6 months for the leuprolide and flutamide group, and 28.3 months for the leuprolide and placebo group; a difference of approximately 25% and a survival advantage of about 7.3 months (p=0.035) (Figure 39). The differences in progression-free and overall survival were more evident in the subgroup of patients with minimal disease and good performance status, and these patients may be the most likely to benefit from combination therapy (Crawford et al., 1989).

Thus, combination therapy produced a small but important improvement in both progression-free survival and overall survival, and the benefits may be greatest in patients with minimal disease. Nevertheless, neither the progression-free period nor overall survival in this study was as great as that claimed by Labrie and associates in their uncontrolled study.

Moreover, several other large double blind studies were unable to detect any difference in median time to progression or survival between patients treated with testicular androgen blockade alone as compared with

PROSTATE CANCER

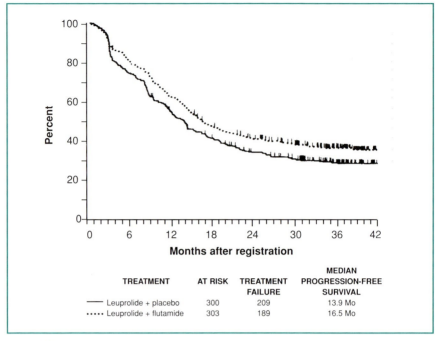

Figure 38. *Progression-free survival.*

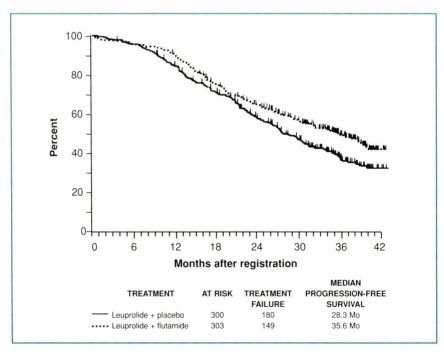

Figure 39. *Overall survival (Two-sided P = 0.035).*

combined androgen blockade. A recent study from Europe with goserelin plus flutamide vs orchidectomy showed delayed time to progression in the total androgen ablation as compared with the orchidectomy group, but overall survival was not significantly different (Denis et al., 1991).

In a prospective study begun in 1986 with 457 patients treated with orchidectomy and then randomized to receive either nilutamide (225 patients) or placebo (232 patients), progression free survival was significantly longer in the nilutamide group (median time to progression 20.8 months in the nilutamide group and 14.9 months in the placebo group; p=0.005). Median time to death was 30 months in the placebo group and 37 months in the nilutamide group.

Objective regressions were higher in the nilutamide group (41%) than in the placebo group (24%). Significant differences in favor of nilutamide were found at several intervals for bone pain, PAP, PAS, alkaline phosphatase and bone scan isotope uptake (Janknegt et al., 1993).

With these conflicting reports on the efficacy of combined androgen ablation, the question remains unresolved. The controversial marginal advantage must be weighed against the side effects of anti-androgens, particularly diarrhoea, and the cost of both drugs.

Perhaps there is a case for combination therapy in the younger patient, with good performance status and low volume disease.

Is early hormonal treatment better than deferred treatment in metastatic prostate cancer?

The issue of whether hormonal therapy should be initiated early or late in patients with advanced prostate cancer has been controversial for some time. The question really applies to patients who are asymptomatic at the time of presentation. Symptomatic patients need to be treated, and few patients with advanced disease (Stage C or D; T3, T4, M1) are asymptomatic at diagnosis.

In a retrospective study, the late Dr Barnes (1981) reviewed the results of 550 of his patients with prostate cancer diagnosed between 1927 and 1972. The 15 year survival of patients with stage A and B tumors who had immediate endocrine therapy was 24% (23/95), compared with 32%

Prostate Cancer

(16/50) among patients given delayed therapy. The decreased survival for patients less than 70 years of age who had immediate therapy was more marked: the immediate-therapy 15 years survival was 35% (17/35), and with delayed therapy it was 46% (11/24). As most of the patients with C and D disease had symptoms when first seen, immediate rather than delayed endocrine treatment was given.

However, a few patients with stage C and D disease who were seen before 1941 (the time when Huggins discovered the hormone dependency of prostatic cancer) and who were still alive at that time were given delayed treatment, resulting in a five year survival of 62% (8/13) compared with the five year survival in patients treated with immediate endocrine therapy of 58% (45/78). The five year survival of those having no therapy was only 23% (3/18).

From these data, Barnes concluded that patients more than 70 years old should not be treated until they have symptoms. Many with stage A and B lesions will never develop symptoms before they die of some other disease or succumb to old age. The study showed that patients given delayed endocrine therapy (no treatment until symptoms appear) have a little better survival than when therapy is started as soon as the diagnosis is made.

This interesting and meticulous study has to be viewed in its historical context. Today, endocrine therapy would not be considered for early localized disease and there is a wider choice of endocrine manipulations for advanced disease than simply estrogens (in dangerously large doses), and orchidectomy.

The VACURG (Veterans Administration Cooperative Urological Research Group) study number 1, carried out during the 1960s, was a prospective, randomized trial that inadvertently addressed the problem of early versus delayed treatment, although it was not designed so to do. The four arms of the study compared:

- placebo
- DES 5 mg
- DES plus orchidectomy
- orchidectomy plus placebo.

About 475 patients were recruited to each arm. The protocol decreed that patients in the placebo arm who showed progression of their disease either by evidence of metastases on X-ray or elevation of PAP could receive endocrine treatment at the investigator's discretion. Thus, the placebo arm was to all intents a delayed endocrine-treatment arm. Since the study included patients with stage 3 (non-metastatic disease), progression from stage 3 to stage 4 could be observed (Figure 40).

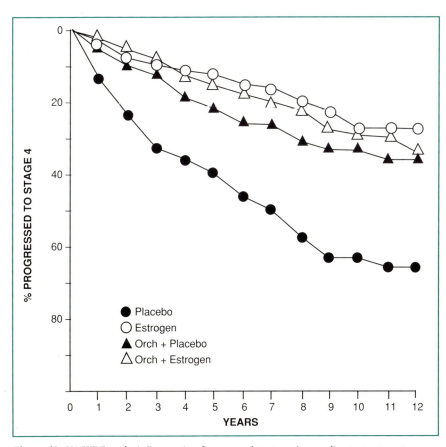

Figure 40. *VACURG study 1. Progression from stage 3 to stage 4 according to treatment.*

It can be seen that in all three endocrine treatment groups, progression was significantly delayed in comparison with the placebo group (Byar and Corle 1988). When overall survival was analysed for the same treatment groups, no significant differences were seen, in spite of the fact that 60% of all deaths were due to prostatic cancer.

These data show that immediate endocrine treatment significantly delays progression of the disease, but there appears to be no survival advantage. It is perhaps wise at this stage to reserve judgement on these findings; they may represent a true picture, but there are a number of unanswered questions. For example, 25% of patients in this study who were treated with DES died from cardiovascular causes.

This vexed question may finally be answered when the results of two prospective studies that are currently in progress become available:

♦ The EORTC, GU group protocol 30846 is a randomized study of patients who at the time of radical prostatectomy are found to have positive pelvic lymph node metastases.

♦ The Medical Research Council of Great Britain is conducting a study into the effects of early versus delayed treatment on duration to progression and survival in asymptomatic patients with metastatic prostatic cancer.

Does hormonal treatment cure prostatic cancer?

Hormonal treatment does not cure prostate cancer. However, about one in ten men with metastatic prostatic cancer receiving palliative hormone therapy will survive for a long period of time (up to ten years) without progression of disease (Reiner et al 1979).

There have also been documented cases of 'cure' in which there was no evidence of residual cancer at autopsy, but these are exceptionally rare (Johansson and Ljunggren, 1981).

If other causes of death do not supervene, all patients with metastatic prostatic cancer will eventually escape from hormonal control and succumb to their disease with an overall median survival of around two years.

What is hormone-escaped disease and why does it occur?

At present, endocrine manipulation is generally accepted as first-line treatment in metastatic disease However, about 20-30% of tumors do not respond at all to endocrine treatment ab initio. Furthermore, in those patients who do respond, remission is transient and after a variable period of time a hormone-unresponsive tumor begins to grow.

What is the mechanism for this relapse phenomenon wherein an initially androgen-sensitive prostate cancer progresses following androgen ablation to an androgen-insensitive state?

The answer to this basic question is critical, since, depending upon the mechanism, it may or may not be possible to prevent or delay the development of such an androgen-insensitive state.

Obviously, like normal prostate development, the hormonal responsiveness of prostatic cancer must correlate with the presence of a normal, or partially normal, functioning of the androgen receptors. In the case of androgen-dependent tumor growth at least one, but most probably more, control mechanisms of the regulation of prostate development must be modified. This might include the androgen-dependent pathway downstream of the androgen receptor and/or one of the as yet unidentified androgen-independent control processes. Unresponsiveness of tumor growth might correlate with the absence of the receptor, the presence of an intact receptor, or the presence of a mutated receptor.

Like the normal prostate, androgen-dependent prostatic cancers retain the requirement of androgen to simultaneously stimulate their rate of cell division and inhibit their rate of cell death. Unlike normal prostatic cells, however, such androgen-dependent prostatic cancer cells have a faster rate of cell division than cell death when sufficient androgen is present, which results in their continuous proliferative overgrowth.

Two plausible explanations for hormone escape have been suggested by Isaacs (1984). One possible mechanism for the relapse to androgen deprivation is that prostatic cancers are initially composed of tumor cells that are homogeneous, at least with regard to their requirement for androgen. Following castration, most of these dependent cells stop proliferating and die, thus producing an initial response to hormonal manipulation. However, some of these androgen-dependent cells randomly adapt under environmental pressure to become androgen-independent. The androgen-independent cells proliferate to re-populate the tumor, producing a relapse after castration.

This hypothesis presupposes that changing host environmental conditions following hormonal manipulation are critically involved in inducing the adaptive transformation of an intitially hormone-dependent to a hormone-independent tumor cell (Figure 41).

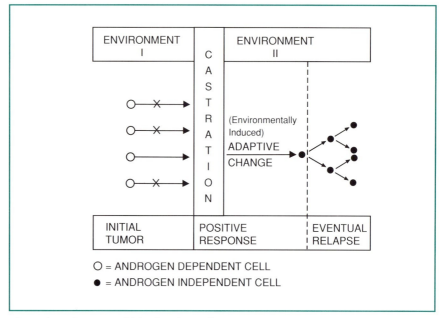

Figure 41. *Adaption model for the relapse of prostatic cancer to androgen ablation therapy.*

An alternative explanation is that prostatic cancers are initially heterogenous with regard to their androgen requirements for growth, being composed of pre-existing clones of both androgen-dependent and androgen-independent tumor cells. In this circumstance, androgen deprivation would result in the death of only the androgen-dependent cells, without affecting the growth of the androgen-independent ones which continue to proliferate.

Even if these androgen-independent cells represented only a small fraction of the original tumor, they would eventually replace any tumor loss due to death of the androgen-dependent cells, but progressively expand the tumor population producing the relapse phenomenon (Figure 42).

The consensus opinion, supported by experimental studies (Isaacs, 1984), is that prostate cancers are composed of a heterogenous population of cells that differ in their requirement for androgen.

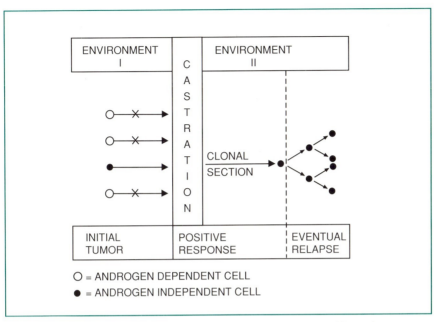

Figure 42. *Clonal model for the relapse of prostatic cancer to androgen ablation therapy.*

Prostatic cancers are composed of clones of cancer cells that are phenotypically heterogenous even before therapy is initiated. There is arguably a case, therefore, for future studies to be directed towards combining androgen ablation plus chemotherapy and/or radiation early in the disease in order to affect both the androgen-dependent and independent cancer cells present in the individual prostatic cancer. It will only be possible to achieve a cure in prostatic cancer when the stem cells of both endocrine responsive and unresponsive clones can be eliminated.

One of the most difficult problems in prostate cancer is what one does for the patient with hormone-escaped disease. Perhaps the first question is to define hormone escape and determine how it can be recognized. The clinician has to rely on biochemical, hematologic, radiologic, radioisotope, ultrasound and clinical changes to arrive at an informed opinion about hormone escape or disease progression.

What are the signs of progression in prostate cancer?

The earliest sign of disease progression will be a rise in consecutive PSA values which tend to pre-empt clinical change. Killian et al., (1985) have shown that the higher the elevated serum PSA concentrations, the greater the likelihood of tumor recurrence, and the shorter the interval to clinical detection of that recurrence.

Prostate Cancer

All patients with a PSA value ≥ 88 ng/ml (40 times higher than normal) had a recurrent tumor, with a mean interval between the elevated serum PSA determination and clinical detection of less than two months. In 92% of the patients, the serum PSA level was elevated before tumor recurrence; the mean lead time between elevation and clinical detection of the tumor recurrence was 12 months.

Does one treat a patient with a rising PSA before the onset of clinical symptoms?

While there is general agreement that a rising PSA is an indication of disease progression, there are no really effective therapeutic alternatives for hormone-escaped or hormone-resistant disease. Most clinicians would be reluctant to embark on second-line treatment until such time as symptomatic relapse, in the form of bone pain, obstructive uropathy or clinical deterioration, was apparent.

CHAPTER FIVE

THE TREATMENT OF HORMONE-ESCAPED DISEASE

What are the treatment options for hormone-escaped disease?

The assumption that hormone-escaped tumor cells are sustained by low levels of residual adrenal androgen encouraged attempts to remove the source of these androgens by adrenalectomy, hypophysectomy, or the drug aminoglutethamide. However, because few patients responded only symptomatically, and then not for long, most of these methods of secondary endocrine treatment have been abandoned.

The synthesis of various alkylating agents with steroids as biologic carriers in the hope that the estrogen would target the drug to the estrogen receptor on the cancer cell appeared to be a novel chemotherapeutic approach. Estramustine phosphate, a water soluble 17-β phosphate of estradiol-3-N-bis (β-chloroethyl) carbamate, was introduced into clinical practice in 1966. It is a molecule in which estradiol and nitrogen mustard are bound together with a carbamate linkage in an attempt to combine their hormonal and cytotoxic actions. Pharmacokinetic studies show that estramustine phosphate is rapidly metabolized to the cytotoxic active compounds estromustine and estramustine.

Estromustine is a steroidal N-mustard derivative, but it has no alkylating or hormonal effects. Estramustine brings about disassembly of the microtubules leading to the disorientation of chromosomes in the metaphase. The compound binds to the microtubule-associated proteins which are essential for microtubule stability. About 10% of the cytotoxic metabolites are hydrolyzed to estrone and estradiol, which produces a depression of total testosterone.

Estramustine accumulates in tumor tissue to a greater extent than in benign hyperplastic tissue. The advantage of estramustine phosphate over other cytotoxic drugs is its ease of administration, tolerance and relatively few side effects. A total of 19 Phase II studies have been performed with

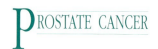
PROSTATE CANCER

estramustine phosphate (650 patients). The objective response rate was 30–35% and the subjective response rate about 60% (Janknegt, 1992).

Other experimental drugs have been studied. The anti-fungal agent, ketaconazole, which suppresses androgen production, has been used, but gastro-intestinal side effects and hepatotoxicity limit its potential usefulness. A related imidazole, liarozole, may have fewer side effects. Suramin, a growth factor antagonist, may also be of some value. These compounds are presently under investigation.

Clinical experience suggests that patients with relapse after endocrine therapy have an average survival time of only 6 months and further endocrine manipulation is of little value. Chemotherapy and radiotherapy then become the only other options.

What is the role of cytotoxic chemotherapy in the treatment of hormone-escaped disease?

Over the past 20 years, several studies have reported the use of various cytotoxic drug regimens for the treatment of hormone-relapsed cases. The results have been discouraging and unrewarding. Clinical experience with chemotherapy is best illustrated in a recent study by the Southwest Oncology Group reported by Wozniak et al., (1993), in which 57 patients who had failed previous hormonal manipulation were treated with a combination of cyclophosphamide, methotrexate and 5-fluorouracil.

There were only two (7%) partial responses and a further ten patients (17%) had stable disease. Median survival was 10.9 and 10.2 months, respectively, for the two groups. Median survival of patients was not dissimilar to that of previous reports in which median survival of patients with metastatic prostatic cancer who failed hormone therapy was 44 weeks.

The toxicity associated with these potent alkylating agents and anti-metabolites in this elderly, often frail and debilitated group of patients can be severe and unacceptable and treatment-related deaths have been known to occur. Cytotoxics appear to have little part to play in the treatment of hormone-escaped prostate cancer.

What is the treatment for painful bony metastases in hormone-failed patients?

Bone metastases are the commonest cause of pain in cancer which results in immobility, pathological fractures, bone marrow failure, neurological symptoms and hypercalcemia. The management of skeletal metastases is directed towards symptom palliation and demands a multi-disciplinary approach. Treatment may involve radiotherapy, oncology, surgery, nuclear medicine and palliative care.

Analgesics

Analgesics form the basis for managing metastatic bone pain. Guidelines for the sequential use of non-steroidal anti-inflammatory drugs (NSAIDS), NSAIDS with weak opiates, and finally strong opiates have been proposed by the World Health Organisation (WHO 1986). The efficacy of analgesics is often enhanced by concurrent administration of tricyclic anti-depressants and phenothiazines.

Radiotherapy

The analgesic effect of radiation for bone metastases has been recognized since the early 1900s but has been supported by relatively few controlled trials. Two techniques are widely used; local field external beam treatment for discrete, localized pain and wide field (hemi-body irradiation for multi-focal disease). Painful bone metastases often respond dramatically to external beam radiation therapy. With a dose of 3000 to 3500 cGy delivered to the site of pain Benson et al., (1982) obtained relief in 77% of patients.

For metastases in vertebras, a single direct field to the affected area should be used, with a generous margin around the lesion, since the tumor is always more widespread than the X-rays suggest. Another common site is the rib cage and here again local irradiation is effective. Involvement of the weight-bearing bones, particularly the femora if osteoblastic in nature, can be treated with irradiation alone. If osteolytic, with cortical bone destruction, then prophylactic internal fixation should be performed followed by irradiation.

Where there are multiple painful skeletal metastases, relief can be obtained by wide-field or hemi-body irradiation. This is a quick and effective way of controlling bone pain. Response is typically rapid, occurring within 24 - 48 hours of treatment and is maintained until death in the majority of patients. Prospective studies have reported pain relief in 73 - 83% of patients treated with a single fraction of 6 - 7 Gy to the upper hemibody and 6 - 8 Gy to the lower body (Hoskin et al., 1989).

60% of patients develop treatment-related toxicity, particularly nausea, vomiting and diarrhoea. A period of intravenous fluids and anti-emetics may be necessary to minimise these toxic effects. Rarely, radiation pneumonitis may be fatal and myelosuppression affects virtually all patients who receive sequential upper and lower hemi-body irradiation.

Strontium-89

The therapeutic potential of the beta particle emitter, Sr-89, was first recognized in the 1940s with the discovery that it was preferentially localized in areas of new bone formation (Pecher, 1942). Strontium, being closely related to calcium in the periodic table, is physiologically treated like calcium and is preferentially taken up by bone and teeth. The radioisotope is given as an out-patient intravenous infusion. There is no risk to family or the public from its urinary excretion unless the patient is incontinent, and then this treatment is inappropriate. Following intravenous injection Sr89 is cleared rapidly from the vascular compartment and selectively concentrates at sites of increased bone mineral turnover.

Biodistribution studies using the gamma emitter 85 Sr in patients with metastatic prostate cancer showed strontium retention at 90 days following injection ranging from 11 - 88% depending largely on the extent of the bone involvement by tumor. Absorbed doses to tumor in the range 20 - 24 cGy/MBq have been calculated giving a therapeutic ratio of metastases to red marrow of 10:1 (Blake et al., 1988).

Pain relief in 75% of patients with disseminated prostatic cancer has been reported. Those with limited skeletal metastases respond better than those with more widespread disease. Reduction in pain and analgesic requirement are achieved in 70 - 80 % of patients, with complete relief of pain in 20% after a single infusion. The time to response is two - four weeks and the median duration of benefit four - six months, so 40 - 50% of patients are likely to remain pain-free until death from advancing disease. Re-treatment has been possible at approximately three month intervals on up to eight occasions with repeated pain relief, but with the risk of cummulative toxicity.

As with hemi-body irradiation, myelosuppression is the main toxic effect - the platelet count may fall to 70% of pre-treatment level within four - six weeks of treatment. Myelosuppression is worse in patients with extensive metastatic disease, especially those with low with pre-treatment cytopenia (Sr89 could prove fatal since three - six months is required for recovery) (Robinson et al., 1987).

Sumarium-153

Sumarium 153 has a shorter physical half-life than the beta emitters and there is a suggestion that Sumarium 153 may be more effective than 89 Sr for the relief of metastatic bone pain. A series of stable S, 153 complexes have been synthesized using multidentate acetate and phsophonate ligands of which Sm 153-ethylenediaminotetramethylene-phosphonate (Sm- 153 EDTMP) has the most favorable in vivo distribution. The radioisotope is stable in vivo and clears rapidly from the blood following intravenous injection. 40 - 60% of the dose is excreted in the urine within eight hours, the remaining activity is concentrated in the skeleton, with preferential uptake at sites on increased osteoblastic activity. Lesion to normal bone uptake ratios of 17:1 have been calculated.

In a recent prospective, randomized, controlled study, Sr89 in a dose of 200 MBq was compared with small field radiotherapy or hemi-body radiotherapy in the treatment of painful metastases. The study showed that Sr89 was as good as external radiotherapy in controlling pain. There was a reduction in the incidence of new sites of pain in those treated with Sr89, and that treatment morbidity was less than those give hemi-body radiotherapy. Because of the reduction in the incidence of new sites of pain, there may be some advantage in giving Sr89 early in the disease, but it does not work for all patients and does not appear to be very effective where there is a pathologic fracture.

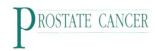

CHAPTER SIX
SCREENING

Should we screen our 'at risk' population for cancer of the prostate?

The term 'screening' needs to be defined. Screening means the testing of all men within the population who meet certain criteria as part of a community health program. It should not be confused with the opportunistic testing as part of medical care for those who seek advice for other conditions. Both practices are becoming increasingly common; one, stimulated by national cancer/urological societies and the other by the opportunistic testing by measurement of PSA.

Due to the low prevalence of the disease in men under 50 years of age and the limited life-expectancy of men over 70, screening, if it is to be undertaken at all, should apply to men between the ages of 50 and 70 years. However, to screen or not to screen for prostate cancer has become one of the most contentious issues in urology in recent times.

The aims of screening for prostate cancer should be threefold:

♦ to improve early detection of the disease
♦ to improve survival from the time of diagnosis
♦ to reduce disease-specific mortality.

To achieve these objectives, it is important to consider the principles for screening that apply to any disease, as outlined by Wilson and Jungner (1968).

1. The condition needs to be common and an important health problem (carcinoma of the prostate is the most commonly diagnosed male cancer in the USA and the second or third most common cause of death in the Western world).

2. The diagnostic tests need to have a high degree of sensitivity and specificity (the three methods used to screen for prostate cancer, i.e. DRE, TRUS and PSA, fall short on all counts).

3. The tests should be easy to perform and interpret and universally available, affordable and repeatable at regular intervals.

4. The screening procedure should be acceptable to the patient.

5. Screening should result in the detection of the disease at a curable stage that will significantly improve the chance of survival.

6. Neither treatment or screening should cause an unacceptable degree of physical or mental morbidity (there is no evidence as yet that screening for carcinoma of the prostate actually reduces mortality from the disease).

Given these criteria, it is not difficult to see why the question of screening for prostate cancer is so controversial.

However, screening programs are already in operation and we need, therefore, to consider their impact on the clinical management and outcome of the disease and on the available resources. Among DRE, PSA, and TRUS, DRE is the most imprecise, with a positive predictive value of around 20%. The entire screening-debate revolves around PSA as the single most important diagnostic beacon.

The probability of prostatic cancer in a patient with a normal prostate on rectal examination and a PSA level below 4 ng/ml is 2.5%; in patients with a PSA between 4 and 10 ng/ml it is 5.5%; and in those with a PSA level over 10 ng/ml it is 30%. Nevertheless, there is a 20–30% false-negative rate in men with localized disease, and a 15–25% false-positive rate.

PSA has a lower probability of error (36%) than either DRE or TRUS. PSA in combination with DRE has the lowest probability of error (56%) of the various double combinations of the three screening tests (Catalona et al., 1991).

The current consensus is that PSA and DRE should be used as the initial screening test, with TRUS reserved for those patients who have abnormal findings in DRE, PSA, or both. Guidelines recently published by the American Cancer Society recommended that men over the age of 50 should have an annual digital examination and PSA assay. This policy is endorsed by the American Urological Association and the US College of Radiotherapists.

Has 'screening' improved the early detection of prostate cancer?

Most of the increase in the reported incidence of prostate cancer is attributable to the introduction of screening for the disease in some countries. The reported incidence of prostate cancer in the United States has shown a dramatic 16% increase in one year, and the number of prostate cancers diagnosed has virtually doubled in the last four years, apparently because larger numbers of men are now having their PSA levels assessed. The incidence will continue to climb in the next few years as more and more countries adopt screening. PSA is easy to perform and there is an indiscriminate readiness on the part of clinicians and, in some cases, a demanding public for the test without weighing the consequences.

It is inappropriate in asymptomatic 75 or 80 year old men. Once done, it is inevitable that some will need a biopsy and a substantial proportion will seek further treatment (Chisholm, 1993).

In a PSA-based screening of 1653 men, prostate cancer was detected in 37 (2.2%). 35 of these underwent a radical prostatectomy, but only 11 had organ-confined disease as determined by pathologic staging (Catalona et al., 1991).

Nevertheless, in this study screening resulted in the diagnosis of 20 times more cases than would have been expected from a reported incidence of approximately 100/100,000.

Screening and opportunistic testing will indeed detect more clinically important tumors at an asymptomatic stage. Approximately one third will be localized, organ-confined carcinomas amenable to curative treatment with either radical prostatectomy or radiotherapy. If TRUS-guided biopsies are performed as part of the screening process, a small percentage of the large number of latent carcinomas will be uncovered.

It is thought that most latent carcinomas cannot be detected by DRE, PSA or TRUS, which explains the disparity between the detection rate with screening and the incidence of latent cancers at autopsy. Two thirds of the cases diagnosed on screening will have either locally advanced or metastatic disease.

Will screening improve survival from the time of diagnosis for patients with organ-confined cancer?

This question cannot be answered at the present time. It will require long-term, randomized, controlled studies comparing radical prostatectomy with radiotherapy and with deferred treatment to answer it. Deferred treatment warrants consideration as a management option because, in a study from Sweden of 223 patients with localized prostatic cancer treated expectantly, the disease-specific survival rate at 10 years was 86.8% (Johansson et al., 1992). This question may be answered more swiftly if the scientific laboratory enquiries that are in progress can identify the malignant potential of prostatic cancers and help us to distinguish the pussy cat from the tiger.

Will screening improve survival from the time of diagnosis for patients with asymptomatic locally advanced or metastatic cancer?

Once again, this question cannot be answered as yet. It will, to some extent, depend upon the results of studies currently being carried to determine whether early versus deferred treatment improves survival. It also begs the question - what treatment?

A factor that needs to be considered in respect of the interpretation of survival data is the 'lead-time bias'. For example, if a man develops prostatic cancer at 51, becomes symptomatic at 61 (when the cancer is diagnosed) and then dies at 64 years of age, his survival time is reported as 3 years from diagnosis. If, as a result of screening, the same man's cancer is diagnosed at 54 and is treated aggressively but he still dies at 64, his survival time from diagnosis becomes 8 years. Thus, there is an apparent improvement in survival although the man has not actually lived any longer. A false impression has been created that screening led to improved survival.

What are the adverse effects of screening on the patient?

Although there are little hard data on the psychological effects of screening on men in this age group, there is inherent a high level of false-positive PSA results, combined with the inaccuracies of DRE and TRUS, a very real potential for harm that may outweigh the benefits. Many of these men will have to undergo a prostatic biopsy, a procedure which carries a risk, albeit small, of infection. In some, a negative result will allay the fear of cancer, but in others the detection of clinically insignificant disease may engender an intolerable degree of psychological distress.

It could also be argued that the morbidity and mortality associated with radical surgery and radiotherapy are unacceptable until such time as randomized, controlled trials show a proven advantage over a wait and watch policy in the management of organ-confined disease. Finally, there is the emotional and psychological trauma of the man who has to live for longer with knowledge of his incurable cancer.

At the present time, no screening studies have been shown to reduce the mortality from prostatic cancer. Although screening programs are in progress in both the USA and Europe, it will be at least ten years before the answers are available.

Prostate Cancer

CHAPTER 7

QUESTIONS COMMONLY ASKED BY PATIENTS – DERMOTT LANIGAN
SENIOR REGISTRAR, UROLOGY, GLASGOW ROYAL INFIRMARY.

How serious is it, doctor?

A significant problem for all doctors who treat cancer is the application of the known determinants of disease outcome to the individual patient. Most prognostic indicators (such as tumor stage and grade), while giving good indications of the behaviour of tumors in patient groups, are less useful in any single case. This is because the clinical course of an individual patient is affected by three factors: the biological properties of the tumor, the response of the host and the effective treatment; as our understanding of all these aspects of cancer biology is incomplete, it is impossible to give a completely accurate prognosis. Furthermore, the issue of the prognosis of cancer of the prostate is clouded by our lack of understanding of its natural history, unresolved debates among specialists about the place of the various options for management and the commercial haze that surrounds some of the options for medical management.

Despite these difficulties, the patient rightly expects his physician to provide an informed and personalised interpretation of his condition, and particularly will wish to know how likely the disease is to do him serious harm. Several factors need to be taken into account in assessing the potential lethality of the cancer.

It is a truism that many more patients die with cancer of the prostate than from it. In one study of early, untreated disease with long term follow up (means 123 months) 56% of patients died, but prostate cancer was the cause of death in only 8.5%. It is not surprising that studies show that intercurrent disease accounts for many more deaths following diagnosis in the mainly elderly population who suffer from this disease. Nevertheless, certain features enable us to make generalizations about those who are likely to do badly.

Prostate Cancer

Patients who have high grade cancer tend to do significantly worse than those with more differentiated tumors, regardless of initial stage of disease or other factors, In other words, grade (commonly expressed using the Gleason System) is an independent prognostic indicator.

Patients who show poor biochemical or clinical response to treatment usually suffer early relapse or progression. In practice, those patients whose PSA levels fall rapidly to normal following treatment have a longer progression-free survival than others. A fall of PSA of <90% is associated with worse outcome. Broadly, it seems also that the PSA level at diagnosis is related to prognosis. Patients with levels of <100ng/dl do better than those with levels >100, with those >500 doing worse again.

Patients in whom disease progression is metastatic rather than local are at higher risk of relapse following treatment. Why some tumors tend to grow extensively around the gland, whilst others metastasise early to bones is unclear, and this behaviour may represent fundamental biological differences in the tumours themselves.

Clinically significant (i.e. potentially lethal) tumors tend to progress in the few years following diagnosis, and, in general, those who survive for 10 years or more do not tend to display late progression.

Poor performance status at presentation has been shown to be an independent indicator of adverse outcome. This is common sense: those patients rendered ill because of their cancer of concurrent illness must be expected to fare worse than patients who are in good general condition at presentation. Bone pain, anemia or elevated alkaline phosphatase are also harbingers of poor prognosis. Black men appear also to have a worse outcome than other racial groups.

While the above represents a series of generalizations, all the factors mentioned have been shown to be independent prognostic indicators. Following on from this, we an expect that the more of these adverse features displayed by an individual, the worse the outlook.

I've had my prostate gland removed so aren't I alright now?

Patients who have had a transurethral prostatectomy and who have been told that the gland was benign are often surprised if they are subsequently diagnosed as having cancer of the prostate. Malignant growths of the prostate tend to begin in the periphery of the gland, which generally is unaffected by TURP. Prostatic zones have been discussed elsewhere, but only a quarter of cancers begin in the transitional zone, which is the zone of origin of benign prostatic hypertrophy, while 67% of cancers occur in the peripheral zone. TURP therefore offers no protection against the development of carcinoma.

Do I have a choice of treatment?

The relative merits and effectiveness of the various treatment options have been covered in the relevant sections. However, it is clear that patient preferences are very important. Many patients, of course, will not have strong feelings about their treatment but younger men, particularly sexually active ones, will wish to participate in the decisions about which treatment suits them best. One of the few studies of patient preference for hormonal manipulation found that, when offered a choice, roughly half of the men opted for orchidectomy, and the others for parenteral LH-RH agonists (oral agents were not included).

Most of the latter group cited the desire to avoid surgery as their main reason. An interesting survey of Norwegian Urologists reported that just over a third would opt for surgery (mainly for the convenience of having a 'once-off' treatment), although two of them wished first to have a trial of LH-RH agonists in order to assess tumor hormone dependence. For many men, (particularly the elderly, those with low-grade disease or even, perhaps, some of those who are afraid of all of the options) a decision to defer treatment, and to monitor their clinical status and the PSA will be entirely reasonable.

Will I need further surgery?

Most patients who have had a TURP will not require a re-do if they have been found to have cancer of the prostate. For those tumors which exhibit local recurrence, adequate control of symptoms can usually be achieved by hormonal treatment (including orchidectomy). A small, unfortunate subgroup will need occasional 'channel' resections.

Radical surgical options will usually be discussed with appropriate patients by the urologist.

Very rarely, orthopedic procedures will be indicated for the complications of bony metastases.

Prostate Cancer

Is a more effective cure on the way?

At the time of writing, it does not appear as if any significant advances are likely in the near future. A lot of research attention is being focused on quality of life issues. The background research for gene therapy in cancer of the prostate is being done, but several significant problems await solution before animal studies of this exciting work can be reproduced in man.

My treatment gives me hot flushes. Can anything be done?

At least two thirds of patients who have had orchidectomy or LH-RH agonists have some trouble with hot flushes. They are caused by the effects of sudden hormone withdrawal on the hypothalamic thermoregulatory centres and catecholamine levels. Effective treatment is readily available.

Medroxyprogesterone acetate, cyproterone acetate or estrogen all provide the required sex-hormone replacement, though the latter drug has the drawbacks of possible cardiovasculare side-effects as well as feminization.

Will I become incontinent?

Aside from the particular side effect of incontinence following radical prostatectomy, very few men with cancer of the prostate will have problems with continence. The exception is that group of men with extensive local disease, in whom the cancer invades the external urinary sphincter. This situation is often accompanied by the development of stress incontinence.

This group of men often have a difficult combination of obstructed voiding and incontinence. They are doubly unfortunate as transurthral resection often relieves the former while making the latter symptom worse. There are several reasons for this. The bulk of obstructing tissue is often an aid to continence in those with malignant infiltration, and therefore weakness, of the sphincter. Debulking the tumor creates a larger channel, and the cancer-infiltrated sphincteric muscle is no longer strong enough to cope.

At operation, it can often be difficult to make out the usual landmarks for the external sphincter in this situation and the urologist tries to strike a balance between creating a sufficiently large channel and avoidance of sphincter damage, as far as possible.

Will the treatment make me impotent?

Radical nerve-sparing retropubic prostatectomy carried out by an experienced surgeon is associated with development of impotence in fewer than 10% of previously potent patients. For radical radiotherapy to the prostate, the quoted figures vary, but may be as high as 50%. Because it does not affect circulating testosterone levels, a pure anti-androgen such as flutamide, when used as monotherapy, helps lower the incidence of impotence in those men who require hormonal manipulation but are keen to avoid impotence.

As outlined elsewhere, there is some evidence that monotherapy (as opposed to complete androgen blockade) may be associated with a somewhat shorter progression-free interval, although the evidence as to whether it is also linked to shorter survival is contradictory. In any case, a suitably informed and motivated patient may be willing to accept the trade-off.

Will hormone treatment cure me?

Not unnaturally, patients who are prescribed powerful drugs with significant side-effects accept the medication in other expectation of 'cure'. The question of cure, like many other aspects of this disease, is not a simple one. Symptoms such as bone pain, those arising from local prostatic tumor and occasionally malaise and weakness often do resolve after initiation of hormone treatment.

However, the duration of response to such therapy is variable and finite with media figures of the order of 18-20 months. As we have seen, the likelihood of a prolonged response can to some extent be forecast by the trend in PSA fall after therapy commences. Sooner or later though, many patients will suffer relapse or progression of their disease.

Could I have done anything/do anything to prevent the disease?

No. Etiologic factors are unclear for this cancer. There is some evidence suggesting a familial component to development, of prostate tumors and the black race is a relative risk factor.

It has also been suggested that promiscuity may have a role, but the evidence is weak. No other lifestyle features have discernible effect on the risks of either development or progression of the cancer. There is also no evidence of a link between vasectomy and this disease.

Prostate Cancer

REFERENCES

Armstrong B, Doll R. (1975) Environmental factors and cancer incidence and mortality in different countries, with special reference to dietary practices Int. J. Cancer: 15: 617 - 631.

Barnes RW, (1981) Endocrine therapy of prostatic carcinoma. In Prostatic Cancer Ed. Richard J Ablin. Marcel Dekker, Inc. New York pp 219 - 228.

Benson RC, Hasam SM, Jones AG, Schlise S. (1982). External beam radiotherapy for palliation of pain from metastatic carcinoma of the the prostate. J. Urol 127: 69-71.

Benson RC (1992) A rationale for the use of non-steroidal anti-androgens in the management of prostate cancer. Prostate (Suppl) 4: 85 - 90.

Berg JW, (1975) Can nutrition explain the pattern of international epidemiology of hormone-dependent cancers? Cancer Res. 35: 3345 - 3350.

Boring CC, Squires TS, Tong T. (1992) Cancer Statistics, 1991 Ca-A Cancer J Clinicians 41: 19 - 37.

Byar DP, Corle DK. (1988) Hormone therapy for prostate cancer: Results of the Veterans Administration Cooperative Urological Research Group Studies. NCI Monographs 7: 165 - 170.

Cantrell BB, DeKlerk DP, Eggleston JC, Boitnott JK, Walsh PC (1981) Pathological factors that influence prognosis in stage A prostatic cancer: the influence of extent versus grade. J Urol.125: 516 -520.

Carter HB, Pearson JD, Metter EJ et al. (1992) Longitudinal evaluation of prostate-specific antigen levels in men with and without prostate disease. JAMA 267 (16) 2215-2220.

Cooper JF, Foti A. (1974) A radioimmunoassay for prostatic acid phosphatase. 1. Methodology and range of normal male serum values. Invest. Urol. 12: 98 - 102.

Crawford ED, Eisenberger MA, McLeod DG, Spaulding JT, Benson R, Dorr FA, Blumenstein BA, Davis MA, Goodman PJ. (1989) A Controlled trial of leuprolide with and without flutamide in prostatic carcinoma. New Engl. J. Med 321: 419 - 429.

Daehlin L, Thore J, Bergman B, Damber J-E, Selstam G. (1985) Direct inhibitory effects of natural and synthetic estrogens on testosterone release from human testicular tissue in vitro. Scand J. Urol. Nephrol. 19: 7 -12.

Denis L, Smith P, Carneiro-de-Moura JL, Newling D, Bono A, Keuppens F, Mahler C, Robinson M, Sylvester, R, DePauw M, Vermeylen K, Ongena P. (1991) Total androgen ablation: European experience. Urol. Clin. North Amer. 18: 65 - 73.

Prostate Cancer

Franks LM (1954) Latent carcinoma of the prostate. J. Pathol Bacteriol. 68: 603 - 616.

Geller J, Albert JD, Nachtsheim DA, Loza D. (1984) Comparison of prostatic cancer tissue dihydrotestosterone levels at the time of relapse following orchiectomy or estrogen therapy. J. Urol, 132: 693 - 696.

Gleason D.F., Mellinger, G.T. (1974) Veterans Administration Cooperative Urological Research Group: Prediction of prognosis for prostatic adenocarcinoma by combined histological grading and clinical staging. J. Urol 111: 58-64.

Gutman AB, Gutman EB. (1938) An 'acid' phosphatase occurring in the serum of patients with metastasizing carcinoma of the prostate gland.
J Clin Invest 17: 473 - 478.

Hoskin PJ, Ford HT, Harmer CL. (1989) Hemibody irradiation for metastatic bone pain in two histologically distinct groups of patients. Clon Oncol 1:67-69.

Isaacs JT. (1984). The timing of androgen ablation therapy and/or chemotherapy in the treatment of prostatic cancer. The Prostate 5: 1 - 17.

Janknegt RA. (1992). Estramustine phosphate and other cytotoxic drugs in the treatment of poor prognostic advanced prostate cancer.
The Prostate (Supplement) 4: 105 - 110.

Johansson S, Ljunggren E. (1981). Prostatic carcinoma cured with hormonal treatment. Scand J. Urol. Nephrol 15: 331 - 332.

Killian CS, Yang N, Enrich LJ, Vargas FP, Kuriyama M, Wang MC, Slack NH, Papsidero JD Murphy G, Chu TM (1985). Prognostic importance of prostatic-specific antigen for monitoring patients with stages B2 to D1 prostate cancer. Cancer Research 45: 886.

Kipling MD, Waterhouse JAH. (1967) Cadmium and prostate cancer.
Lancet 1: 730 - 731.

Kramer SA, Spahr J, Brendler CB, Glenn JF, Paulson DF (1980) Experience with Gleason's histopathological grading in prostatic cancer. J. Urol. 124: 223 - 225.

Labrie F, Dupont A, Belanger A, Lacoursiere Y, Raynaud J, Husson J, Gareau J, Fazekas A, Sandow J, Monfette G, Edmond J, Joule G. (1983) New approach in the treatment of prostate cancer: Complete instead of partial withdrawal of androgens. Prostate. 4: 579 - 594.

Leman RA, Lee JS, Wagoner JK, Blejer HP. (1976) Cancer mortality among cadmium production workers. Ann NY Acad Sci. 271: 273 - 279.

Lund F, Rasmussen F. (1988) Flutamide versus stilboestrol in the management of advanced prostatic cancer. Br. J. Urol. 61: 140- 142.

Lundgren R, Sundin T, Colleen S, Lindstedt E, Wadstrom L, Carlsson S, Hellsten S, Pompeius R, Holmquist B, Nilsson T, Rubin S, Luttropp W, Jansen H. (1986). Cardiovascular complications of estrogen therapy for non-disseminated prostatic carcinoma. Scand. J. Urol. Nephrol 20: 101 - 105.

McNeal JE. (1984) Anatomy of the prostate and morphogenesis of BPH. in new approaches to the study of Benign Prostatic Hyperplasia. Alan R Liss Inc., 150 Fifth Avenue, New York NY 10011: pp 27-53.

Melner MH, Abney TO, (1980) The direct effect of 17 bioestradiol on LH-stimulated testosterone production in hypophysectomised rats.
J. Steroid Biochem 13: 203 - 210.

Mostofi FK, Sesterhenn IA, Davis CJ. (1992) A pathologist's view of prostatic cancer. Cancer (Suppl) 71: 906 - 932.

Neumann F. (1983) Pharmacological basis for clinical use of anti-androgens.
J. Steroid Biochem 19: 391 - 402.

Papas AA, Gadsden RH. (1984) Prostatic acid phosphatase: Clinical utility in detection, assessment and monitoring carcinoma of the prostate. Annals of Clinical and Laboratory Science 14: 285 - 291.

Pecher C. (1942). Biological investigations with radioactive calcium and strontium: preliminary report on the use of radioactive strontium in the treatement of bone cancer. Univ Cali Publ Phamocol 11:117-149.

Peeling WB, (1989) Phase III studies to compare goserelin (Zoladex) with orchiectomy and with diethylstilbestrol in treatment of prostatic carcinoma Urology. (Suppl) 33: 45 - 52.

Peto R, Doll, R, Buckley JD, (1981) Can dietary beta-carotene materially reduce human cancer rates? Nature 290: 210 - 208.

Redding TW, Schally AV. (1981) Inhibition of prostate tumor growth in two rat models by chronic administration of D-Trp analog of luteinizing hormone-releasing hormone. Proc. Nat. Acad. Sci. USA 78: 6509 - 6512.

Reiner WG, Scott WW, Eggleston JC Walsh PC (1979). Long-term survival after hormonal therapy for stage D prostate cancer. J. Urol 122: 183 - 184.

Roberts JT, Essenhigh DM. (1986) Adenocarcinoma of prostate in a 40 year old body-builder. Lancet 2: 742.

Prostate Cancer

Robinson RG, Spicer JA, Preston DF, Wegst AV, Martin NL. (1987) Treatment of metastatic bone pain with strontium-89. Nucl Med Biol 14: 219-222.

Rooney C, Beral V, Maconochie N, Frase P, Davies G. (1993) Case control study of prostatic cancer in employees of the United Kingdom Atomic Energy Authority. Brit. Med. J. 307: 1391 - 1397.

Ross RK, Paganini-Hill A, Henderson BE. (1983) Epidemiology of prostate cancer. In Urological Cancer. Ed. Donald G. Skinner. Grune & Stratton. New York. pp 1-19.

Ross RK, Bernstein L, Lobo RA, Shimizu H, Stanczyk FZ, Pike MC, Henderson BE. (1992) 5-alpha reductase activity and risk of prostate cancer among Japanese and US white and black males. Lancet. 339: 887 - 889.

Sagalowsky AI, Milam H, Reveley R, Silva FG. (1982) Prediction of lymphatic metastases by Gleason histological grading in prostatic cancer. J. Urol. 128: 951-952.

Schroder FH. (1993) Endocrine therapy for prostate cancer: Recent developments and current status. Brit. J. Urol. 71: 633 - 640.

Schroeder HA, Nason AP, Tipton, IH. (1967) Essential trace metals in man: zinc relation to environmental cadmium. J. Chronic Dis. 20: 179 - 210.

Scott WW, Schirmer HKA, (1966) A new oral progestational steroid effective in treating prostatic cancer. Trans. A, Assoc Genitourin. Surg 58: 54 - 60.

Sogani PC, Whitmore WF. (1979) Experience with flutamide in previously untreated patients with advanced prostatic cancer. J. Urol, 122: 640 - 643.

Stamey TA, Kabalin JN, Ferrari M, Yang N (1989). Prostate specific antigen in the diagnosis and treatment of adenocarcinoma of the prostate. 1V Anti-androgen treated patients. J Urol. 141: 183A.

Wilson JMJ, Jungner G. (1968) Principles and practice of screening for diasease. WHO Public Health Paper: 1 - 34.

Winkelstein W, Kantor S. (1969) Prostatic cancer - relationship to suspected particulate air polution. Am J. Publ. Health 59: 1134 - 1138.

World Health Organisation (1986) Cancer pain relief. WHO, Geneva.

Wozniak AJ, Blumenstein BA, Crawford ED, Boileua M, Rivkin SE, Fletcher WS, (1993) Cyclophosphamide, methotrexate and 5-fluorouracil in the treatment of metstatic prostatic cancer. A Southwest Oncology Group study. Cancer. 71: 3975-3978.

ACKNOWLEDGEMENTS

Table 3. *The Limits of Surgery in the Cure of Prostatic Carcinoma.* European Board of Urology.

Figure 6. *British Journal of Urology.* Churchill Livingstone Ltd.

Figures 13 and 14. *Manual of transrectal ultrasound of the prostate gland.* Schering-Plough.

Figure 17. *Difficult diagnosis in urology.* Churchill Livingstone, Inc.

Figure 24. *Mechansims of progression to hormone independent growth of breast and prostatic cancer.* Parthenon Publishing Group Limited.

Figure 26. *Drug Therapy of Prostatic Cancer.* Adis International Ltd.

Figure 29. *Adjuvant Endocrine Treatment of Prostatic Cancer.* EBU Education Committee by Royal Society of Medicine Services Ltd.

Figures 30 and 31. *Estracyt – Scientific Edition 2.* Pharmacia Leo Therapeutics AB.

Figures 38 and 39. *The New England Journal of Medicine.* Massachusetts Medical Society.

Prostate Cancer